PRESCRIPTION FOR TOTAL HEALTH AND LONGEVITY

by

Jonas E. Miller, M.D.

with

Jason Vinley

Logos International
Plainfield, New Jersey

PRESCRIPTION FOR TOTAL HEALTH AND LONGEVITY
Copyright © 1979 by Logos International
All rights reserved
Printed in the United States of America
Library of Congress Catalog Card Number: 79-83523
International Standard Book Number: 0-88270-353-6
Logos International, Plainfield, New Jersey 07060

To the host of God's children
who need to know how best to care for
God's temple—the human body—which houses
both soul and spirit.

———————

And the very God of peace sanctify you
wholly; and I pray God your whole spirit
and soul and body be preserved blameless
unto the coming of our Lord Jesus Christ.
(1 Thessalonians 5:23)

CONTENTS

FOREWORD

Jonas E. Miller, M.D. brings forth a much needed ministry to the body of Christ—that of dealing with the total man: spirit, soul and body. Spanning more than five decades as a practicing physician, counselor and ordained minister of the gospel, his life eminently qualifies him to write this book.

Born in 1900, Dr. Miller has an incredible witness—he has never had a confining illness all his adult life. This is even more outstanding when one realizes the thousands upon thousands of sick bodies and minds he has helped to heal in his lifelong practice. Dr. Miller still commands a full medical clinic in Sarasota, Florida, with a large staff working under him. He lectures an average of one hundred times per year to both churches and professional organizations.

Dr. Miller is, above all, a man of compassion who wants to share the practical application of the time-proven truths he has compiled through years of ministry and medical studies that you might live a fuller, more abundant life.

Throughout his rich, robust life, Dr. Miller has led a balanced existence. He has conducted camp meetings, medical seminars, evangelistic meetings, and has lectured on health and physiology before thousands of both professional and nonprofessional groups. He has written articles for both religious and medical publications, and has served as staff contributor and editor for several magazines including *Successful Living Magazine* and *The American Journal for Medico-Physical Research*. During his lifetime he has pioneered five different churches which are still flourishing today.

In the earlier years of his career he lived in Washington, D.C., where he was medical director for the Health Foundation with fourteen aides working under him. Simultaneously, Dr. Miller pastored Calvary Gospel Church and taught and served as dean at Bethel Bible School. During this period he also had a national radio program on healthful living over the Mutual Broadcasting System. He is a graduate of Baltimore Medical College and a member of the National Medical Society, the International Academy of Preventive Medicine, the National Hospital Association, the Florida Naturopathic Medical Society, the American Association for Medico-Physical Research, and is the founder and current secretary of the American College for Studies in Metabolism and Endocrinology.

The above listing of degrees and honors is only partial, because Dr. Miller continues to pursue knowledge and understanding in both fields to which God has called him, as a minister of God's Word and a physician. He lives by a maxim, "You do not grow old. When you stop learning, you are old." It is out of this proven and tried life of scriptural understanding and medical knowledge that he brings forth *Prescription for Total Health and Longevity* that you might live a healthier, fuller life spiritually, emotionally and physically in the midst of these complex times.

PRESCRIPTION FOR TOTAL HEALTH AND LONGEVITY

WHY THIS BOOK WAS WRITTEN

"I don't understand you, Dr. Miller," a well-intentioned, middle-aged sister in the Lord said to me one day. "I've heard you preach. I've seen the Lord use you to heal the sick through prayer. I've listened to you teach on divine healing many times. Why don't you just quit your medical practice and preach the gospel?"

"Listen," I replied, wondering if Luke, the beloved physician, ever had such a confrontation with God's people, "I believe in divine healing more than you do!"

"How can you say that? Why, I wouldn't even take an aspirin for a headache, and you give medicine to people all the time."

"I can say it because I'm not as disposed to sickness as you are right now."

"What do you mean?" she asked me, suddenly looking very sheepish.

I explained that in all probability my body's "immune system" was much stronger than hers, because I observed God's natural laws for health which I knew she didn't. Fortunately, she became a patient of mine shortly thereafter and began to observe some of the truths I've written in this book. This conversation took place over thirty years ago, but I've seen the healthful change in this dear woman's life which has allowed her to lead a happier, more abundant life in the service of the Lord.

Many Christians today are bound by the same dilemma which they interpret as a conflict between faith and knowledge. Throughout my life I've had to defend my faith in God's healing power simply because He called me to be a physician. Faith and knowledge are not at odds with each other any more than grace and works are or any other seeming paradox of the Bible. I once had a friend who said, "If you think science and the Bible conflict with each other, it's because you don't know enough science, or you don't know enough Bible." And I believe that's true.

I have faith in God to heal anyone according to His Word. I have seen it happen many times. I've prayed for people to be healed, and I've seen the omnipotent hand of the Almighty touch and deliver people from many sicknesses and infirmities. Yet at the same time I also have faith to allow God to use me as a doctor and to minister to the sick through my knowledge of His "natural laws" and medical science.

One of the reasons for this book is expressed by Hosea, "My people are destroyed for lack of knowledge" (Hos. 4:6). And literally, so many of God's people today are being destroyed simply because they have very little or absolutely no knowledge of how to maintain their own emotional and physical well-being. They have every fine intention of pursuing the things of God by studying His Word, praying and having fellowship, but when they are confronted with their physical nature, or taking care of their bodies and minds, they somehow categorize this as "worldliness" or an aspect of their old, fallen nature. They don't realize God made them total human beings—spirit, soul and body (1 Thess. 5:23); and that He wants them to "be in health, even as thy soul prospereth" (3 John 2).

But the truth is that many Christians suffer today because they simply mistreat their bodies and don't know they're doing it. Many people say to me, after I show them they can alleviate their ailments by changing their diets or instructing them in the proper order of eating, "My, I didn't know that. I didn't realize the way I was eating was causing me to get sick." And I say, "Well, that's what Hosea said. You're destroying yourself because you just don't know."

For too long there have been those in the church who have spiritualized every aspect of being to the extent that they want nothing to do with knowledge of God's natural laws of health or medicine. Yet the Scriptures say, "A merry heart doeth good like a medicine" (Prov. 17:22). Obviously medicine or medical knowledge must have a benefit for us. Paul referred to Luke as the "beloved physician" (Col. 4:14). The Bible also makes it clear that many great men of God became sick at different times in their lives, notably Trophimus (2 Tim. 4:20), Timothy (1 Tim. 5:23), Epaphroditus (Phil. 2:25, 26) and Paul (Gal. 4:13, 14). Even Elisha, a man who was given a "double portion" of the Spirit and worked tremendous miracles for the Lord, fell sick and died (2 Kings 13:14, 20).

God has made us tremendously complex creatures, and it is for us to marvel at His glorious construction in our lives. "You made all the delicate, inner parts of my body, and knit them together in my mother's womb. Thank you for making me so wonderfully complex! It is amazing to think about. Your workmanship is marvelous—and how well I know it" (Ps. 139:13, 14 TLB). There are times when medical knowledge can relieve a physical ailment. There are other times when only prayer can save a person's life. I have seen them both. Yet it is no marvel to me that the Lord said, "It is the sick who need a doctor, not those in good health" (Luke 5:31 TLB).

I remember as a young boy reading the story of Solomon in

3

the Bible. God gave him the opportunity to ask for whatever he wanted. Because he didn't ask for selfish things like long life and riches, but asked for "a wise and an understanding heart" (1 Kings 3:12), God granted his request. This story touched me so much that I bowed my head and told God I wanted knowledge so that I could help people who were in trouble. This happened when I was eleven years old. My life has been a testimony to that answered prayer.

As a physician I have delivered babies. As a minister, I then dedicated them to God. I prayed for them when they needed that too. I have seen these same babies grow into men and women and give their hearts to the Lord. I baptized them and accepted them into the church. When they wanted to marry, I filled out their blood tests as a physician and married them as their pastor. Then during times of crises, I have spent some long vigils at their bedsides until they passed from earth into eternity. In those sad cases I filled out their death certificates as a doctor, and preached their funeral sermons as a minister.

My life has been a rich and full one shared with a wonderful Christian wife and four children who are all grown and living for the Lord. I've had the honor of preaching God's Word in some of the finest churches in the land, and I've had the opportunity to care for diplomats, members of congress and of the cabinet, and have been invited to two presidential inaugurations. In all these things I give God the glory for the truly marvelous grace He has shed upon me in my professional life as a doctor and an ordained minister of His Word.

I've always tried to be obedient to God's leading. I've learned that whenever you're honest with God and honest with yourself, He will grant you the desires of your heart (Ps. 37:4). The problem with most people is that they're not honest with God because they don't know how to be honest with themselves. Often they smother themselves in religious platitudes and traditions of men, thinking it's the "right thing to do" or "how to act," and they never let go and get real with God. Their minds are confused by trying to imitate some other brother or sister in the Lord, instead of truly becoming like children and taking everything to their Father in simple, childlike faith and believing for their real needs and desires no matter how foolish some of these needs might seem to their carnal minds. The key is *honesty*.

In 1949, I felt the Lord impressing me to give up my flourishing medical practice in Sarasota, Florida, and go into full-time ministry. As a doctor with an established practice, I was making a very good living; and I was truly being blessed on every hand. I was active in Christian work, was raising a family and prospering in the profession God had given me the ability to practice. Yet I knew the Lord was moving me into a new realm of obedience to Him, and I couldn't resist the urging of His Spirit. So I sold my practice and did what I felt was the honest leading of God in my life. I'm not saying it was easy, but down in my innermost being—in what the Bible calls my "heart"—I was being honest with myself and with God. So I left all behind for the gospel's sake.

For approximately five years from 1950 to 1955, I worked in full-time ministry. I taught the Word of God at a well-known Bible college in the Southeast and helped promote that school for nearly two years. Then for the next three years I was involved in full-time evangelism and teaching across the United States. It was during these evangelistic and teaching sessions, held in various churches throughout the nation, that I really started to minister to the "total man"—spirit, soul and body.

It all came about while I was ministering in a series of meetings at Aaron Wilson's large church in Kansas City, Missouri. Back in the fifties it wasn't uncommon to hold a series of meetings for two or three weeks at a time, and I was

5

scheduled to have the meetings in his church for a full two weeks, beginning on Tuesday night. They did not schedule services for Monday evenings because most people would not attend so soon after Sunday.

As the services got under way the first week, I asked Aaron if it would be all right with him if I would minister on the care of the mind and the body in the light of the Scriptures on the coming Monday night. He said he didn't mind but warned me that nobody would come out on a Monday night. He told me about a situation that occurred just several months earlier. A very famous evangelist was holding some meetings in the church and made the mistake of having services on a Monday night when hardly a soul showed up.

I told him I understood the odds were against me, but I had wanted to minister on the topics of the mind and body for some time. So on Friday night I announced that the Monday night service would deal with scriptural teaching about care of the mind and body. There was no further publicity. Well, it turned out that more people came to hear me on Monday night than any other night. In fact, we drew a bigger crowd on Monday than we did on Sunday!

This dramatized the fact to me that God's people really wanted to know about healthful living in all areas of life—spiritually, emotionally and physically. From that point on I would always ask host pastors if I could do the same thing. They usually agreed and the results were always the same. The people came out in good numbers to learn. Soon I conducted two meetings on the same topics; one night would involve the care of the mind, and the other night, the care of the body. After these meetings people would come up to me and ask, "What kind of book could you recommend for us to learn more?" Others would inquire, "Haven't you written a book on physical and emotional health that we can get?" I would have to tell them

I was sorry, and explain that I hadn't written such a book. But I had always intended to do just that if and when I found the time for such a task.

Finally, I was able to sort out all the notes, tapes and case histories and knit them together into a meaningful, practical book for God's people to prosper from and enjoy. For, you see, it was in 1955, at the end of that full-time ministry in my life, that God audibly spoke to me and gave me new direction for my life.

My wife, Elizabeth, and I had arrived in Dallas, Texas, in August for a series of meetings only to discover there had been a split in the church, and the meetings had been cancelled. Remembering that "all things work together for good to them that love God" (Rom 8:28), I decided to call ahead to Fort Worth where I had scheduled meetings two weeks later. To my shock I was informed that that church's pastor had just resigned, and they had cancelled my meetings too!

Four weeks later, I was scheduled to speak in Oklahoma City. Seeing our predicament, I decided to call ahead to learn if there was some way they could have the meetings before the scheduled dates. Although the pastor sympathized with our plight, he informed us that this was the middle of August and they were experiencing one of the worst heat spells they had ever had. He guaranteed that the people wouldn't come out in such torrid conditions. This was before air-conditioned churches were popular. So there we were—stuck in Texas for six weeks with nothing to do. Finally we decided to drive to Waxahachie, Texas, where we knew some friends from Bible school. I can remember how hot it was because when we walked down the asphalt roads in the noonday sun, we could actually slide on the pavement.

When we arrived, we found a little motel. To our delight it had air-conditioning. We decided to stay there for a while and wait on the Lord for direction. My wife and I began to fast and pray for God's guidance in our stranded situation. We literally didn't know which way to turn or where to go next. In the evenings we visited many of the different tent meetings around the countryside in those days. During the day we stayed in our cool room to fast and pray.

After we were there five days, the Lord spoke to me in a dream. It was so vivid, and His voice was so real; I shall never forget it. It was as if the Lord were sitting in the room with me. He said, "You have proven yourself. Go back to your work. Obey me, and I'll make up to you everything you have ever sacrificed for the gospel."

I immediately awakened and shared the dream with Elizabeth. After we talked and prayed some more, we decided I had indeed heard the Lord speaking and that we should be obedient to His direction. After years in full-time ministry, traveling across the forty-eight states, I stopped my evangelistic meetings and returned to Sarasota, Florida, to reopen my medical practice which I had left five years earlier.

I've been fulfilling this call of God on my life ever since and He has been faithful to His spoken word. He has given more to me than I ever gave to Him during those five years of ministry.

I still run a medical clinic with a full staff of technicians. Solomon said, "there is no new thing under the sun" (Eccles. 1:9). This confirms that we learn from each other. In my fifty years of professional experience I have attended many medical seminars where I have learned from others. What I learn I process in the crucible of my own life and practice. In the past two years I have attended twenty-two such professional seminars on endocrinology, metabolism, nutrition, vitaminology, holistic medicine, geriatrics, immunology, hormone therapy and other related subjects. I have tried what I feel is good for my patients; in many instances I use myself as a "guinea pig." In this book I report on only those things which I have personally proven to be beneficial to me or my patients.

This continuous research throughout my professional life has taken me around the world twice, to Europe eight times, and on visits to sixty foreign countries. I have also shared this information with hundreds of physicians in teaching seminars I have led in this country and abroad. I have discovered there is a trend of going back to the basics of life and nature. More and more natural methods of healing, diet and health are being rediscovered or used in conjunction with some of the marvelous methods of modern medicine.

My entire life has been spent in learning about God, and God's favorite creature, man. "It is the glory of God to conceal a thing: but the honour of kings is to search out a matter" (Prov. 25:2). I'm not a king, but as Harold Hill, a Spirit-filled engineer and scientist, has put it, "I'm a King's kid!" Since I've been a King's kid most of my life, it's been an honor to search out the manifold wisdom of God both in the spiritual and physical realms. That's what this book is about. My heart's desire is to bring to God's people some of the knowledge He has allowed me to discover that they may lead healthier, wholesome lives as "total" men and women.

I know some of the principles in this book will seem controversial to some and revolutionary to others, but I also know that the results of applying these principles and teachings have helped me to live a full life in which I can honestly testify I've never had a confining illness during all of my adult years, in spite of the fact that I treat thousands of sick people every year and I'm constantly in contact with illness and disease. Believe me, my intention has never been to be controversial, but simply to share the truth as I have learned it. My hope is that this book will help consummate Paul's prayer for the body of Christ, "I pray God your whole spirit and soul and body be preserved blameless unto the coming of our Lord Jesus Christ" (1 Thess. 5:23).

THE REAL YOU

Man's spiritual hunger can never be satisfied apart from God. Man's total healing can never be fully accomplished apart from dealing with his spiritual nature.

Jesus once asked a man, "Wilt thou be made whole?" (John 5:6). He was referring to physical healing. But there are many places in the Bible where the Lord made contact with people, and they were made whole emotionally, spiritually and physically. Jesus is interested in the total person. He wants us to be whole. He wants us to be total human beings, for He was totally man and totally God. Throughout the Scriptures we find Him referred to as the Son of Man and the Son of God, and He cares for us in every aspect of our beings.

It's important that we notice the order in which wholeness is to come to us (1 Thess. 5:23). This Scripture tells us "your whole spirit and soul and body"—in that precise order. Not, as many people today use the phrase, "body, soul and spirit." In God's set of priorities it's your spirit that comes first because "God is a Spirit: and they that worship him must worship him in spirit and in truth" (John 4:24). You can't worship God unless it's in the spiritual realm. You can talk about Him. You can think about Him. You might even write great theological treatises about Him, but the only way you can worship Him is in your spirit, because God is a Spirit. That's why He considers your spiritual nature most important when dealing with your total being.

Until your spirit finds union with God through Jesus Christ, you will always be spiritually hungry. You may not recognize the symptoms of spiritual hunger, but they are there. I'm a physician, and I've learned to recognize malnutrition when I examine a patient. Even though the initial appearance seems to be okay, a thorough examination reveals the patient is suffering from malnutrition because he is lacking vital nutrients in his body. Unless this need is taken care of, the person will eventually die.

In the same way spiritual malnutrition will cause a person to die before his time. The signs of spiritual hunger are really quite evident if you look for them. The spiritually hungry person who is without Christ will seek to satiate himself in worldly pleasures or counterfeit spiritual endeavors. By worldly pleasures I mean a craving for things that appeal to what the Bible calls the "carnal" or "natural" man—things like movies, television, travel, novels, amusements, etc. Now all these are all right when they are used in moderation. But the spiritually hungry person will find himself seeking these areas and similar ones to an inordinate degree, because he's seeking spiritual fulfillment but doesn't know how to find it.

By counterfeit spiritual endeavors I mean false religions and occult practices. Since our nation has been inundated with a host of these belief systems within the last decade, I'd like to relate my personal experience involving a man who has promoted belief in a very definite counterfeit spiritual experience—that of reincarnation. His name is Edgar Cayce.

Edgar Cayce was a noted psychic. Although he died several years ago, many books have been written about his "life readings'' and predictions. He has literally influenced thousands in our country to believe in the Hindu concept of reincarnation. Cayce gave these "life readings" during a hypnotic state, a form of trance. When he was giving one of these readings to a person, he would claim to take the individual back to a previous lifetime. While thus learning of actions in previous lifetimes, the person would supposedly learn why certain situations and developments were affecting his present life. Hence, the person discovered what the Hindus call his "karma."

Karma is the belief that the soul perpetuates its own destiny based upon the ethical acts it performs from lifetime to lifetime. Each supposed lifetime gives the person an accumulation of either good or bad karma until eventually that soul doesn't have to be reincarnated any more. There is no concept of sin and the judgment of God since the person will work out his own karma for good or bad in the next incarnation. Therefore the concept of a definitive heaven and hell is totally ignored by people who believe in reincarnation. They claim heaven and hell are here on earth now, and that each person experiences them based upon his degree of good or bad karma.

Edgar Cayce was my patient back in the 1930s, while I was working with another physician in Virginia Beach. I examined and treated him for a back and shoulder problem from which he had been suffering for some time. Mr. Cayce was a very pleasant man, and during the course of treatments we had several very interesting conversations. He told me about his belief in reincarnation and the "life readings" he gave for people. He was very sincere in what he believed, but because I was a born-again Christian who knew God's Word, I couldn't believe such an unscriptural concept.

Yet one day when he offered to give me a "life reading" free of charge, I must admit that my interest was piqued. Not that I could ever bring myself to believe in such an untenable position, but I might discover how he was convincing so many people to believe in this spiritual counterfeit, for at this time he had already established quite a local reputation.

Edgar Cayce told me I had lived in at least two other lifetimes. In one I was a great musician in the Old World. In the other I was supposedly a very prominent man who worked by making things out of metal and steel. Now it was all very interesting, and as I said, Mr. Cayce was a very sincere man who believed in what he was doing, but I would like to assure you that there is no such thing as reincarnation. I discovered two very good explanations for the phenomenon that Edgar Cayce performed while in his trance state: one comes from the scientific study of genetic memory, and the other involves a comparison with similar proceedings that occurred in the Bible.

Genetic memory is simply a term used for the biological study that deals with heredity or the genetic composition of an organism. I've been able to help people nutritionally by discovering their genetic background and having them alter their diets accordingly. This is discussed in another section of this book. All genetic knowledge is passed from one person to another descendant in his same line. It's inherited and subconsciously stored in the body's total system, in your genes. Our genetic information goes back ultimately to Adam through all of our ancestors. From time to time we experience situations or events that seem to draw from our genetic memory unexplainable feelings, thoughts or reactions. Let me give you an example.

During World II my son was stationed in Germany with the military. While he was there, he shipped me a phonograph record he had found. It contained certain songs and children's choruses from that land. Now I have been able to trace my ancestry through several generations of Germans, but at this time in my life I had never been to the old country. I had never seen or heard the pealing of church bells that echo through some of those ancient valleys along the Swiss-German border from where my people originated. I had never heard children singing like this before. Yet when I played it, there was something that welled up within me as if I had heard it all before, and I was tremendously moved. I believe that something in my genetic background was touched very deeply. It couldn't have just been the quality of the music, because for someone who didn't have my genetic lineage, it probably wouldn't have had the same effect.

Years later, when I actually had the opportunity to visit the land of my ancestors, there were moments when I actually could foretell what would be up ahead in a place before I arrived. I could be driving along a mountain road, and I knew and could actually visualize in detail what would be around the bend as if I had been there before. Invariably, I would be right. Yet I had never been there.

You've probably experienced the same type of sensation some time in your life. You've said, "Somehow I feel as if I've been here before." This is known as *déjà vu*. You know you've never been there before, but somewhere in your genetic line your ancestors may have been there, and the genetic information they absorbed through their lives has been passed down to their descendants through their genes. When conditions and stimuli are right, the stored information springs forth.

After Mr. Cayce gave me a life reading, I decided to find out as much as I could about my ancestry. Coming from a long line of Amish-Mennonite people who for years lived and worked peaceably among themselves without marrying outside of their group, it wasn't too hard to do.

I was able to trace my roots all the way back to Samuel Miller who emigrated from Canton of Berne, Switzerland, to

Philadelphia, Pennsylvania, in 1763. Then I discovered in my ancestry that in the European town where my people had lived for nearly three centuries there lived a very notable musician of his day. Edgar Cayce had said that in one lifetime I was a famous musician in the Old World, and here it was—the knowledge that there was a famous musician in my ancestry! I believe Mr. Cayce—in his hypnotic state—was able to pick up this genetic information from my subconscious and from that, he inferred that I was a musician in a previous lifetime.

In the second instance he said I had been a prominent metal worker. I found that in my family tree many years ago in America, there was a man who lived among my people who was known as a great man with metals. People would come from miles around to get him to make axes, knives or other hardware, and he prospered in his craft. Of course, I was not that person, but Mr. Cayce had tapped the genetic information in my subconscious mind and asserted that I was.

I once delivered a lecture on genetic information at New College in Sarasota, Florida, and the Counsel-General of Switzerland was present. After I had given this explanation, he came up to me and said, "That is the best explanation of reincarnation I have ever heard." But there is another explanation that may be less scientific. Nonetheless, it is quite direct, and I use it as supportive evidence to show that there is no such thing as reincarnation. This approach comes from the Word of God.

One of the biggest reasons people get ensnared with psychics like Edgar Cayce is because much of what these people say or predict does come true. As I mentioned earlier, man's spiritual hunger will either drive him into materialism or counterfeit spiritual experiences, unless he finds Christ. The devil knows man's frailty and the human desire to know things beyond his limited senses, so he sets up spiritual happenings that will prove to be true in order to trap individuals. If something is 99 percent true and 1 percent wrong, it's still *wrong*. With God, His Word is always 100 percent true.

God warns His people in both the Old and New Testaments about people who divine the future. Psychics like Edgar Cayce, who placed himself in a trance to delve into supernatural matters, are not only twentieth-century phenomena. Astrologers, witches or other so-called "occult sciences" are not only particular to our day either. The Lord named them all back in the book of Deuteronomy and told us how He felt about such people. "There shalt not be found among you any one . . . that useth divination [foretelling the future by any occult means], or an observer of times [astrologer], or an enchanter [one who goes into a trance or uses trances on others, such as a hypnotist], or a witch or a charmer, or a consulter with familiar spirits, or a wizard, or a necromancer. For all that do these things are an abomination unto the Lord" (Deut. 18:10-12).

God knows—because He created you—that your spiritual nature will seek for spiritual experiences through such means when you stop seeking Him. The fact that many who practice these things are able to reveal information about the past or the future that is partially true does not make the seers true prophets. Their ultimate intention is to lead you away from the God of the Bible into a false belief. Listen to this warning, "If there is a prophet among you, or one who claims to foretell the future by dreams, and if his predictions come true but he says, 'Come let us worship the gods of the other nations,' don't listen to him" (Deut. 13:1 TLB).

Edgar Cayce spoke some truth while he was in his trance state, but the ultimate outcome was to lead people away from a belief in the God of the Bible to worship the gods of Hinduism from which stems the belief in reincarnation. It's interesting to note too that Edgar Cayce was teaching Sunday school at a Presbyterian church while he was doing this! I believe Cayce had opened himself up to a "familiar spirit" or a "spirit of divination." Paul cast out such a spirit from a girl in the sixteenth chapter of Acts, and this same kind of spirit used Cayce's mouth and vocal chords to speak lies about reincarnation.

Unfortunately, Edgar Cayce is only one of many different occult personalities popular today, and I single him out only because I knew him personally. But today our newsstands are filled with books and magazines by other psychics, astrologers and fortune tellers all claiming to tell you the truth about yourself, or about the future. It's happening simply because man's spiritual hunger longs to be satisfied. If he won't accept the truth, it will be like this Scripture, "Because they received not the love of the truth, that they might be saved. And for this cause God shall send them strong delusion, that they should believe a lie" (2 Thess. 2:10, 11).

At the beginning of this chapter I mentioned that in God's order of priorities your spirit comes first. Perhaps now that you are a little more aware of some of the spiritual deception so prevalent today, you might understand why God says, "I the Lord thy God am a jealous God" (Exod. 20:5). He is jealous over you. He cares about your spirit, soul and body—your total personality; but essentially your spirit must be whole before total healing will manifest itself through your body and mind because "God is a Spirit."

It is God who created the world as we know it and perceive it. He created it of himself, by himself and for himself. As it is written, "All things were made by him; and without him was not any thing made that was made" (John 1:3). "For by him were all things created, that are in heaven, and that are in earth, visible and invisible" (Col. 1:16). Everything we sense in the material realm was created by God. He literally spoke everything into existence, and it all became material reality. In the first chapter of Genesis, the story of creation, we read the same expression repeatedly: "And God said. . . ." By His supernatural Word He spoke this universe into existence. "Through faith we understand that the worlds were framed by the word of God, so that things which are seen were not made of things which do appear" (Heb. 11:3). The world in which we live is not the result of things we see, but God spoke this visible realm into existence out of His invisible, spiritual realm. The invisible became visible by the Word of God!

An artist creating a picture is a good example of this. We look at the painting and marvel at its beauty. But before it became that colorful display of oils on canvas, it was an idea in the invisible mind of the artist. The same is true of a carpenter building a chair or an architect building a house. Before something material comes into existence, it is first a reality in the invisible mind, and out of that invisible reality, the material creation comes into being.

You were created out of the invisible mind of God. You have been created in the image of God (Gen. 1:26). The phrase, "in God's image" means man was created with the nature of God in him; that is, man was created with a spiritual nature because God is a Spirit. After the fall of man, sin began to destroy the human's spiritual life source, but I want you to notice the details of how real life began: "God formed man of the dust of the ground [his body with no life in it yet] and breathed into his nostrils the breath of life [God's Spirit]; and man became a living soul [a thinking, feeling human being with the ability to make decisions]" (Gen. 2:7). It was the Spirit of God who gave life to man. Before that man was not alive. So when we say we are created in the image of God, it means we have a spiritual nature. It is by this spiritual nature that our physical (body) and emotional (soul) well-being is or should be controlled. God never intended for us to function purely on our physical levels or our emotional (thinking, feeling) levels. Instead he wants these two levels of our being to be led by our spiritual nature. "For as many as are led by the Spirit of God, they are the sons of God" (Rom. 8:14).

I'd like to give you my old physician's definition of death. They don't teach it this way in medical school, but nonetheless, this is how I diagnose death. Solomon said, "There is no man that hath power over the spirit to retain the spirit; neither hath he power in the day of death" (Eccles. 8:8). And I believe that dissolution at death takes place in this manner: God takes His Spirit from the body; the soul, which is the seat of your will, goes to the place prepared for it, heaven or hell, based upon its willful acceptance or rejection of Jesus Christ; and the body returns to the earth, the chemical elements of which it is composed. Like I said, you won't find that definition taught in medical school, but it's true. This is why I always maintain that true healing for the total man or woman always begins in the spiritual realm, just as real life does.

The real you is a spirit! Job said it this way, "Thine hands have made me and fashioned me together round about. . . . Thou hast clothed me with skin and flesh, and hast fenced me with bones and sinews" (Job 10:8, 11). The real Job was clothed with a physical body: skin, flesh, bones and sinews. Spiritually he was a reality in the image of God before the Lord gave him a body. So were you.

This real you is what Paul was referring to when he spoke of the "inward man." "Though our outward man perish, yet the inward man is renewed day by day" (2 Cor. 4:16). The outward man is the physical body; the inward man is the real you. Paul prays for the church, "Be strengthened with might by his Spirit in the inner man" (Eph. 3:16). The "inner man" is the same as the "inward man." Peter refers to the real you as "the hidden man of the heart" (1 Pet. 3:4). All these references refer to the spiritual man within you—"the inward man," "the inner man," or "the hidden man of the heart." It is this invisible man, the spiritual man within your body, that must draw all its strength from God the Spirit to activate all your physical and emotional well-being and to bring total healing to your body and soul.

The real you won't die when your physical body dies. You'll be no less a person when you die than you are when you're physically alive. Isn't this why Jesus said so emphatically, "And fear not them which kill the body, but are not able to kill the soul" (Matt. 10:28)? You will live forever. This is the gospel message. There is life after death. You will continue to exist in the place of your own choosing—heaven or hell.

Let me illustrate this fact from two other passages of Scripture. In Luke 8:49-55, we read the account of the death of the synagogue ruler's daughter. Jesus goes to the ruler's house and tells everybody she isn't dead at all. They had all witnessed her death and were mourning for her. When Jesus said she wasn't dead, "they laughed him to scorn knowing that she was dead." But Jesus commands her back to "physical" life, and we read, "And her spirit came again, and she arose straightway." Her body had ceased to function. It was dead, but her spirit was alive. When her spirit entered her body again at the Lord's command, physical life resumed. The real girl, that "inward man" had simply left her body. But she was alive!

Then in Luke 16:22-26, we find the story of the beggar Lazarus and the rich man. They both died physically, and Lazarus went to heaven (the bosom of Abraham), while the rich man went to hell. Yet they continued their conversation even though they had both died upon the earth! They continued to exist, one in heaven and the other in hell. Incidentally, there can't be a clearer refutation of reincarnation than this passage of Scripture. When you leave your body, you're not going to come back to this earth again; you're going to be in one of two very distinct places, heaven or hell. Yes, the real you will live after you die. No wonder Paul could say so joyfully, "For to me to live is Christ, and to die is gain" (Phil. 1:21). No wonder he could write that magnificent chapter on the Resurrection in the fifteenth chapter of 1 Corinthians. He knew, "There is a natural body, and there is a spiritual body" (1 Cor. 15:44).

Too many people in the medical profession today minister only to the physical body. Sometimes this is unavoidable because of time and other limitations. Frequently, this is what the patient needs.

Whenever possible, I try to minister to my patients "totally." I've found by asking questions about their lives, their needs, and then listening to them talk, I am more able to accurately diagnose their conditions and prescribe remedies for them. So often their problems are all tied up together—physical, emotional and spiritual. When possible, I try to tap the true source for their healing—the real source of life, in the spirit of my patients. Otherwise I know I'm only scratching the surface of an iceberg.

Sarah Kofsky was a case in which this approach worked. Sarah, a Jewish girl, confessed she was an atheist. This was the source of much of her trouble because she was denying her real self, her spiritual nature. She was operating on purely physical and mental levels like so many people today, because she hadn't become spiritually alive. So in addition to the necessary medicine, I prescribed that she read a portion of the Bible every day. At first she remonstrated against me for meddling in her affairs, but I handled this by telling her I was the physician and she was the patient. Reluctantly, she followed my advice. In a short period of time this led to her receiving Christ as her

Messiah! She found Jesus and gave her heart to Him who is alive forevermore and experienced peace for the first time in her life! Peace—what greater remedy is there for so many of today's ills? Sarah testified of this, and my joy was later deepened when I had the privilege of baptizing her.

Yes, I had ministered medicine to Sarah for her physical condition, but it was her spiritual rebirth that brought about the beginning of total healing in her life. And because of it she is leading a happier, fuller, richer life today. This is why I am so emphatic in saying that all true healing begins in the spiritual realm. When you experience spiritual rebirth through Jesus Christ, you literally link yourself with the source of all life—the God who created you in the first place. "But he that is joined unto the Lord is one spirit" (1 Cor. 6:17). Without this vital source a person will continue to function only in the physical and mental levels of existence. Spiritually he will be lost and without access to the source of real life. "He that hath the Son hath life; and he that hath not the Son of God hath not life" (1 John 5:12).

Do you have life—real life? Do you have spiritual life pulsating through your body and mind? Do you have this free gift of salvation that is yours for the asking? Have you made Jesus Christ the Lord and Savior of your life? If you're not sure, I would encourage you to settle this question first before you read more of this book.

In the next chapters I've written some very practical and time-proven methods gleaned from my more than fifty years of medical practice to help you both emotionally and physically. As you examine these truths, remember it is your spirit that needs to come alive through salvation in Jesus Christ to bring about your total healing and the restoration of the real you, your "inner man."

The word "salvation" in both the original Hebrew and Greek

means more than just being saved from our sin. As important as that is, salvation has a fuller connotation of deliverance, prosperity, help, victory, safety and *healing*. And it's all yours for the asking. Jesus Christ is not a dead Savior. He is alive! And His power and salvation is available to you now, if you'll invite Him to come into your life. Believe me, this is the best remedy I could prescribe to anyone, and if you want total health and longevity, I'd like you to repeat the following prayer with me.

Heavenly Father, in the name of Jesus I come to you. I believe Jesus died on the cross for my sins and rose again for my salvation. I open the door of my heart now and ask Jesus to come into my life as Savior and Lord. Amen.

If you have confessed that prayer with your mouth and believed it in your heart—deep down in your spirit—the Bible says you are now saved (Rom. 10:9). That means you have received the gift of salvation. And as I said, salvation has all the benefits of deliverance, prosperity, help, victory, safety and *healing*. The real you has come alive for both now and forever! You have tapped the source of all life and healing through your spiritual rebirth. Let's now discover how by your spirit you can begin to control and heal your mind, your emotions and your physical body to live a more abundant life through total healthful living.

3

YOUR NATURAL MIND

Your natural mind is God's worst enemy. "What do you mean by that, Dr. Miller?" some of you are probably asking. "How can my mind be God's enemy? God gave me my mind, and I thought He wanted me to use it?"

The answer is yes, He wants you to use your mind; but He doesn't want it to use you!

Few people today realize how they allow their minds to be instruments against themselves. Instead of learning to channel their minds into the creative, life-giving processes God intended from the beginning, they allow the tyranny of thoughts to dominate their lives. Christians are not exempt from this plight until they begin to take authority over their thoughts and bring their minds into subjection to their spirits as the Scriptures clearly teach. They allow every thought that comes down the pike to play havoc with their peace and joy without ever stopping to "think" whether the thought comes from God, the devil or acid indigestion. By not distinguishing the source of these thoughts, they foolishly claim them as their own; and that's when the problems begin. They allow their minds to dominate them, instead of allowing their reborn spirits to dominate their minds.

When you were born again, you were reconciled to God and your spirit became one with His. "But he that is joined unto the Lord is one spirit" (1 Cor. 6:17). You're linked with God, and you've become a new creation in Him (2 Cor. 5:17). Because of this momentous rebirth of your true identity, your spiritual nature, God wants your spirit to now have dominance over your body and your mind, instead of allowing your body and mind to dominate your spirit. Your life comes under new management. No longer are you to be subject to the lusts of your flesh (Gal. 5:24), or to walk "in the vanity of your mind" (Eph. 4:17). Your spirit was reborn when you accepted Christ, but your mind has to be renewed. Your mind wasn't reborn any more than your body was at your conversion.

Paul says, "The carnal mind is enmity against God: for it is not subject to the law of God, neither indeed can be" (Rom. 8:7). A dictionary definition of enmity is "deep-seated unfriendliness; hostility." That's the way God views your natural, carnal mind with all of its problem-solving ability and rational processes. Your natural mind is still hostile toward God, because it functions only on the principle of deductive and inductive logic, making no provision for the spiritual reality of God. It's like a computer in this manner. And this world doesn't feed your computer with the thoughts of God. That's why God says, "The foolishness of God is wiser than men" (1 Cor. 1:25), and it's also why your natural mind is God's worst enemy. It doesn't think the way He does. "For my thoughts are not your thoughts, neither are your ways my ways, saith the Lord. For as the heavens are higher than the earth, so are my ways higher than your ways, and my thoughts than your thoughts" (Isa. 55:8,9).

Since your mind has not been reborn, it has to be renewed. That's a process that takes some time, but it begins the moment you begin to walk in the Spirit. "And be renewed in the spirit of

26

your mind'' (Eph. 4:23), Paul writes to the Ephesian church. To the church at Rome he wrote, "And be not conformed to this world: but be ye transformed by the renewing of your mind" (Rom. 12:2). God doesn't want you to think like the world thinks any longer. He doesn't want you to be conformed to the thought processes that dominate man in this world system. He doesn't want you to feed your computer with the everyday thought patterns that permeate our media, our educational systems, our government and other sources. No, He doesn't want you to be conformed to those old ways of thinking, but He wants you to be "transformed by the renewing of your mind."

4

METHODS OF RENEWAL

God wouldn't tell you to renew your mind unless He provided specific ways for this to be done. With God's Word and by His Spirit, you have the power. You can renew your mind. Your thoughts no longer need to control you, but you can begin to control them. There are several ways in which this process of renewal takes place, but I would like to discuss five proven methods I have gleaned from the Word of God over the years. These will help you to think more positively and lead a more productive, fulfilling existence.

The Word

The Word of God is "the sword of the Spirit" (Eph. 6:17), and it "is a discerner of the thoughts and intents of the heart" (Heb. 4:12). Nothing will bring about the altering of your thought processes and the renewing of your mind more than the Word of God. It is the primary source in this renewal process. It will let you know immediately where the thoughts you are entertaining at any given moment are coming from; it discerns them and reveals the true intentions of your heart.

God literally means what He says, and His Word can be depended upon more than anything else. It provides comfort, edification, guidance, assurance, faith, strength, encouragement, peace, happiness, teaching and love to mention only a few of its attributes. God's Word brings life. That's why Jesus said, "The words that I speak unto you, they are spirit, and they are life" (John 6:63). Spiritual words—wonderful words of life—will breed new vitality in your thinking processes. Although volumes could be written on the importance of God's Word in a believer's life, and millions of testimonies could be given on how it has changed individuals' thinking, it cannot be said better than the way Solomon put it in the book of Proverbs: "My son, attend to my words; incline thine ear unto my sayings. Let them not depart from thine eyes; keep them in the midst of thine heart. For they are life unto those that find them, and health to all their flesh" (Prov. 4:20-22). That's how God's Word will affect you. It will be health to all of your flesh, and that includes your mind.

In another passage, God gave Joshua a command for successful living: "This book of the law shall not depart out of thy mouth; but thou shalt meditate therein day and night . . . for then thou shalt make thy way prosperous, and then thou shalt have good success" (Josh. 1:8). That word "meditate" means not only reading the Word of God with your conscious mind, but getting it down into your spirit. "In his law doth he meditate day and night" (Ps. 1:2). If you want to renew your mind, it's imperative that you get God's Word deep down in your spirit. Later on when we talk about believing as a mind-renewal process, you'll see how important it is for both the mind and the spirit to function together to alter your emotions, your thoughts and your circumstances by true believing. Meditate upon God's Word.

Prayer

In addition to reading the Word of God, prayer is perhaps the next most important tool in renewing your mind. In fact, it's more than a tool; it's a mighty weapon to use against the dark thoughts with which the enemy of your soul would like to invade your mind. We know that "the whole world lieth in wickedness" (1 John 5:19), and that we're in the world; but prayer is a way of shielding us from the world's vexations. It's one of the ways we wrestle against the "principalities, against powers, against the rulers of the darkness of this world" (Eph. 6:12). You're no longer to conform to the world's system, but God wants you to start redirecting your mind—controlling it instead of letting it control you by the thoughts which the devil and the world would try to put into it. Prayer helps to do this. But it's important to understand here that there are two types of praying. There is praying with the "understanding" (the conscious mind), and there is praying with the spirit.

Praying with the "understanding" is what Paul refers to in 1 Corinthians 14:15. It's the type of praying with which most people are familiar. It's praying with your conscious mind. It's petitioning God for needs and waiting for the answers to come.

You can't have peace while you're worrying. You can't have faith while you're doubting. God wants you to have peace continually by taking every worrisome thought and doubt to Him in prayer so that peace can rule in your mind. Wouldn't you like to have a mind that doesn't worry? Well, that's promised to you through this type of prayer. "Don't worry over anything whatever; tell God every detail of your needs in earnest and thankful prayer, and the peace of God, which transcends human understanding, will keep constant guard over your hearts and *minds* as they rest in Christ Jesus" (Phil. 4:6, 7 Phillips). Literally, God doesn't want you to worry about anything. It's that simple. Jesus said, "Come unto me, all ye that labour and are heavy laden, and I will give you rest" (Matt. 11:28). Rest. Peaceful rest from the cares of this life, the worry, the doubts and the fears. These are the things that plague our minds, and God has given us this wonderful provision through conscious prayer to keep our minds as they rest in Christ Jesus.

Praying in the "spirit" is the other type of prayer God has provided for His children to relieve some of the mental pressures of life and help renew their minds. Praying in the spirit or worshiping in the spirit is mentioned in various passages throughout the New Testament, but we get an exact definition of what that is when we read, "For if I pray in an unknown tongue, my spirit prayeth" (1 Cor. 14:14). Praying in the spirit is what the Bible calls praying in an unknown tongue.

It's called that, because while you are praying in this manner, your conscious mind doesn't understand the language you are praying. The only way anyone understands this language is if the Holy Spirit gives the gift of interpretation of the unknown tongue (1 Cor. 12:10) in a public meeting which is the proper manner for group fellowship. As far as your private devotions go, however, when you're praying in an unknown tongue, you're praying the perfect prayer out of *your spirit directly to God;* and He's the only one that understands you. It by-passes all of your mental processes. "For he that speaketh in an unknown tongue speaketh not unto men, but unto God: for no man understandeth him; howbeit in the spirit he speaketh mysteries" (1 Cor. 14:2).

When you're praying in an unknown tongue, the real you—the hidden man of the heart or your spiritual man—is praying as the Holy Spirit gives the utterance. It's spirit to Spirit. This prayer language could be the language of another nation or it could be an angelic language (1 Cor. 13:1), but in either case the person praying doesn't understand it with his carnal reasoning. He is not praying out of his conscious mind. This unknown tongue is emanating out of the inward man and not his carnal reasoning. Jesus prophesied of this when he said,

"He that believeth on me, as the scripture hath said, out of his belly [inner depths] shall flow rivers of living water" (John 7:38). When this happens, your spirit is praying and your mind is allowed to rest. The Holy Spirit moves upon you to pray, and it is not a conscious, rational process; though you can control it by your conscious mind (1 Cor. 14:27, 28). It is not the same as going into some sort of trance and losing control of yourself, but it is allowing the Holy Spirit to have His way through you by an act of your will.

When you permit this blessed gift to flow through you your mind is allowed to rest, while God's perfect prayer is prayed through you and for you! "In the same way the Spirit comes to the aid of our weakness. We do not even know how we ought to pray, but through our inarticulate groans the Spirit himself is pleading for us, and God who searches our inmost being knows what the Spirit means, because he pleads for God's people in God's own way" (Rom. 8:26, 27 NEB). Isn't that beautiful? God, our Father, is so aware of our limitations that He provides an Intercessor to help us pray, the Holy Spirit.

Probably in no other area of your walk with the Lord will you find the conflict of the natural mind resisting the wooing of the Holy Spirit more evident than when it comes to the issue of praying in an unknown tongue. My own testimony reflects this so clearly.

After graduation from medical school and during the first years of my medical practice in Washington, D.C., I was totally a materialist. This was so even though I was a Christian. I had been born again before I entered college; but by the time I was through, I had been so inculcated with rationalism that unless something could be proven to me scientifically, I would not believe it. Although I said I believed the Bible, I was beginning to doubt it, or at least portions of it. I could accept the morality taught in the Word, but as far as the supernatural manifestations in the life of a believer, I was a skeptic. My carnal mind could not accept these aspects.

I had a patient who reported to me that his wife had been healed at an evangelistic meeting being conducted at a church in the city. I didn't pay much attention to this until several weeks later I saw an ad in the paper that announced this same meeting. My curiosity was aroused and I convinced one of my technicians, a man named Menno Yoder, to accompany me.

I was on the defensive from the moment I entered the church, because the first thing I saw was a woman preacher. This was totally against my upbringing and training which had told me women were to keep silent in the church and that was that. When she opened her mouth to preach, I sat there with my open Bible, ready to dissect everything she said. But to my surprise, everything was scripturally correct. Not only was she preaching the Word of God, but she preached it with such an anointing and vibrancy that I was compelled to listen. Then, as the service progressed, I noticed the informality and the warmth of the people around me. They would raise their hands to praise the Lord. My knowledge of Greek told me that worship meant "to stretch the hands toward" and here these people, who were not Greek scholars, were doing exactly that.

I felt very uneasy, to say the least, and was anxious to leave, but Menno wanted to stay. He walked up to the altar after the service and began to talk to the people and ask them all sorts of questions. He came back to me and reported on what he discovered and we discussed his findings. He said he had heard people groan and chatter and wanted to know if that might be the "dying of the old man," as someone expressed it. I told him I would have to have time to evaluate all of what we saw and heard, which I proceeded to do during the next weeks.

After we left that meeting, I had no intention of ever returning. I showed Menno a textbook on clinical psychology that pointed out how many women lead frustrated emotional lives and usually have to find some sort of expression, often ending up as religious fanatics. Since there were more women at the altar than men, I said we were probably witnessing a form of fanaticism. I didn't know at the time that a group of these "fanatic" women had begun to pray for us, and their prayers kept drawing us back to that meeting night after night, even though our carnal minds would tell us we shouldn't go.

At the end of one service, a child who was brought in with braces on his legs was prayed for and healed. The moment they took those braces off and the boy began to walk, the entire audience was on its feet praising the Lord. I could no longer see what was going on, so I got up and started forward to investigate. In the meantime Menno was coming to tell me about it. We met about halfway down the aisle where there was a man with his hands lifted toward God speaking perfect German. I can still see Menno's face written with amazement as we both stared at each other.

Because my people were Amish, I knew German perfectly and understood what the man was saying. I knew in my heart that this was something supernatural yet I went back to my seat and sat down. I quickly bowed my head and told God that if He was really speaking to us, He would allow this man to come to us so we could talk to him. As I lifted up my head, that very same man stood right in front of me with an outstretched hand! I felt as though he were looking right through me, and I turned to avoid his gaze momentarily. Satan told me immediately that this was nothing supernatural but that the man was speaking his native German tongue. I decided to find out. I started to ask him all sorts of questions about his background and education. I must admit that I was dismayed to find out that his name was Green; he had no German relatives or knowledge of the language he spoke just a few minutes earlier, and was raised in the hills of Virginia.

"Cap'n," he said, "I'm a-tellin' you—they says I don't even talk good English. You see, I ain't never had no schoolin', for my daddy up and died two weeks after I started school and I had to go to work. But I has the gift of speakin' in tongues. I don't know what I says, but it feels awful good inside."

He then asked me if I "heard" him speak in a tongue a little while back. I told him that I had heard him and understood what he said. He began to jump up and down like a boy with a bicycle and called everyone around to come and hear what he said. I tried to argue with them that the term "unknown" was in italics in 1 Corinthians 14 in their Bibles. This meant that in the original Greek that word wasn't there. But it didn't make any difference to Mr. Green or the others. I told them that they didn't understand, but Mr. Green pointed his finger directly in my face and said, "You is the guy that don't understand. You need the Holy Ghost; then you'll understand!"

I was as frustrated as I could be. My mind could not comprehend it, yet deep down, I felt as though it was something supernatural. I had been taught that when I was born again I had received the Holy Spirit. Now I kept remembering Mr. Green pointing his finger at me and saying, "You need the Holy Ghost, then you'll understand." I decided to investigate further.

I went to the Library of Congress and dug up every book I could find on the subject of "speaking in tongues" or "glossolalia" as it's termed in Greek. I actually neglected my medical practice to find out what I could. I had a critical spirit, but I was honest. And when you're honest with God, even though your guard is up, God will meet you more than halfway. After more than two weeks of researching the subject, I became convinced that the experience of receiving the Holy Ghost was real and so was the manifestation of speaking in an unknown tongue.

One night I went back to the church where the meetings were still in progress. After the service, under great conviction, I made my way to the altar. For the first time in many years, I started crying. Satan told me that if any of my patients could see me now, they would surely think I had lost my mind; but I replied, "I don't care what they think. I'm going to that altar." When I got to the altar, someone ushered me into the prayer room where we knelt by a chair in the corner. I was still in tears as I prayed, "Lord, I don't know what I need or what I want; but I'm undone, and I want what you have for me."

Suddenly, I felt a wind blowing over me, and I opened my eyes to see what door or window might be open. None was—I was facing the corner of the room. This wind began to get hot and I turned my face to prevent it from burning me. About this time I felt electricity come through my head and down my arms. The wind seemed to get stronger, so strong that I couldn't hold onto the chair any longer. Next thing I knew, I found myself on the floor. Then I heard the Lord speak. He asked me to put my career on the altar; then he called for my church, my family, and finally, I felt as though I had to crawl on the altar myself. Then God opened the windows of heaven, and waves of His love flowed all over me. I saw Jesus, the Holy City, and millions in darkness needing the gospel of Christ. I was also conscious of hearing myself speaking in a strange language. This kept up for at least two hours. Finally, I was told nearly everyone had gone, and it was time to leave. I found that I could hardly walk at first. I was able to understand why the disciples were thought to be drunk on the day of Pentecost. This experience happened over forty years ago. It was the beginning of a Spirit-filled life which is as rich today as it was back then.

I've related all this to you because I want you to understand how your carnal mind, like mine did, will always strive against the supernatural movings of God. Remember, the Bible says your carnal mind is enmity against God (Rom. 8:7). Speaking in tongues or praying in the spirit is a supernatural gift God has for you if you will yield that rational, natural mind of yours to Him. Your experience will not necessarily be the same as mine but believe me, God has given you a supernatural method of prayer that will help you renew your carnal mind day by day.

Another remarkable thing about praying in the Spirit is that it is the only gift of the Holy Spirit that is given to us whereby we might be built up in the inner man. All of the other gifts of the Holy Spirit (1 Cor. 12) are given for the edification of the church. But praying in an unknown tongue is the one gift that is given to *you* for your personal edification. "He that speaketh in an unknown tongue edifieth himself" (1 Cor. 14:4). God wants you to be spiritually strong. There is no better way to strength than using this gift He has provided for you.

It is a way of bringing your natural mind into subjection and allowing God to have His perfect way with you spiritually. He searches out your innermost, heartfelt needs and desires that can't even be expressed with your conscious mind, and prays the perfect prayer through your spirit. "The spirit of man is the candle of the Lord, searching all the inward parts of the belly" (Prov. 20:27). Remember, we're talking about the renewal of your mind. We're talking about God's provision for this. If you don't take God at His Word and act upon it, then the fault lies with you. It's the same in any area of your walk with the Lord. He doesn't force His ways upon any man, but once you accept them and believe them as truth, He can begin to work. When you pray in an unknown tongue, you are simply taking God at His Word and asking the Holy Spirit to pray for you in the name of Jesus. You're fulfilling this promise, "And these signs shall follow them that believe . . . they shall speak with new tongues" (Mark 16:17). You will be by-passing your natural mind when you do this, but you will begin to understand this passage: "But ye, beloved, building up yourselves on your most holy faith, praying in the Holy Ghost" (Jude 20).

This refreshing method of prayer should become part of your daily devotions. As you're going about your daily routines, sing praises unto God. You'll find yourself quite naturally, and very often, beginning to pray in a special prayer language. It will bless you. It will edify you. Now in the beginning of this new method you may often find that your carnal mind is still thinking or receiving thoughts that such praying isn't doing you any good. The enemy of your soul might inject some thoughts that it is foolishness or even fanatical. But don't listen to these thoughts at times like this. Yield all to Jesus and rebuke the thoughts; then allow God to have His way with you, for you, and through you. Remember, we're not interested in listening to the carnal mind; but we're interested in renewing it.

This is the way Paul prayed. This is the way the Lord wants you to pray—with your understanding and with your spirit. "For if I pray in an unknown tongue, my spirit prayeth, but my understanding is unfruitful. What is it then? I will pray with the spirit, and I will pray with the understanding also" (1 Cor. 14:14, 15). Your mind will be renewed as your spirit is edified.

Channeling Your Mind in New Directions

The Word of God sheds some additional light on the renewing of your mind by telling you that you can direct or channel your thoughts to good things instead of bad things. There's no way you can become a habitually positive, happy child of God if you allow your mind to absorb a steady diet of newspaper headlines, gossip talk shows on television, illicit literature and movies. It's amazing how many Christians will indulge in such works of the devil, and then wonder why they don't have the joy of the Lord and the peace of God keeping their minds. You are accountable to God. Every day of your life, you make decisions. The decisions you make today affect your tomorrows. You are accountable for the decisions you make. You are accountable for the thoughts you permit to fill your mind.

The Bible tells us, "Abstain from all appearance of evil" (1 Thess. 5:22). Jesus so boldly said that if we saw something that was offensive to our eye, it would be better for us to pluck our eye out than to continue watching that evil thing and go into hell (Matt. 5:29)! Contrariwise, God promises to "Keep him in perfect peace, whose mind is stayed on thee" (Isa. 26:3).

How do you keep your mind on God? How do you channel it? It's not by walking around looking up to heaven all day long. No, it's by filling your mind with godly thoughts and refusing entry of all devilish ones. You direct your mind to dwell upon positive thoughts, good thoughts, and train it to reject every negative, evil thought that would try to gain entrance to your mind. "Finally, brethren, whatsoever things are true, whatsoever things are honest, whatsoever things are just, whatsoever things are pure, whatsoever things are lovely, whatsoever things are of good report, if there be any virtue, and if there be any praise, think on these things" (Phil. 4:8). *You* are to do the thinking. You are to make the decisions about the directions in which you will channel your mind. God tells you what type of thoughts to think, but He gives you the responsibility to make the decision to obey Him.

I know some of you have allowed your minds to become so cluttered with negative thoughts and emotions that you wonder how it's possible to direct your mind to think like the passage from Philippians 4:8. It seems nearly impossible, but it's not. Remember, your mind isn't born again; it's being renewed. Day by day as you begin to apply some of these principles from God's Word, you're going to see changes in your thought processes. After a short time you'll be able to instantly recognize negative, depressing or evil thoughts and realize they are not to control you; but you, by the Word of the Lord and His Spirit will be able to control them! Your mind has no right to control you. You have the authority and the means to control it! Your greatest power is the power of choice, and you've already exercised that power in choosing to read these pages. Make no mistake about it; it can be done.

The devil's prime arena is the arena of your natural mind. There's truth to the old saying: ''An idle mind is the devil's playground.'' But there's a greater truth that the church is waking up to today. By using the spiritual weapons of God, we can clean up our playgrounds of the mind and leave no ground for the devil. When you enter God's realm of the Spirit, the devil doesn't have a chance.

''For though we walk in the flesh, we do not war after the flesh: (For the weapons of our warfare are not carnal, but mighty through God to the pulling down of strongholds:) Casting down imaginations, and every high thing that exalteth itself against the knowledge of God, and bringing into captivity every thought to the obedience of Christ'' (2 Cor. 10:3-5). These are strong words. They are militant words. You don't make a negative thought captive by sitting down to have supper with it. You don't coddle it. You cast it out! You throw it down! You take it captive by fighting it with the weapons of the Spirit and slam it into obedience!

Have you read where Jesus said, ''The kingdom of heaven suffereth violence, and the violent take it by force'' (Matt. 11:12)? He wasn't talking about the physical heaven we'll know when we die. No, He was talking about the kingdom of heaven within our hearts and minds today. That's where He wants to reign! When you are bombarded by thoughts of darkness coming from invisible, evil spiritual forces, you have to stand in the armor of God and wield the sword of the Spirit, which is the Word of God (Eph. 6:17). You must say, ''That thought is not of God and in the name of Jesus I rebuke it!'' Then replace it with the written Word of God by speaking it into your mind and heart. That's what it means by taking the kingdom of heaven by violence.

This is not always necessary, but God wants you to channel your mind to think on the good and lovely things He has made. Before you can do that, you have to war against evil thoughts that would try to invade your mind and take control. The point is this: don't allow your mind to dwell on the wicked thoughts that vie for your attention in this world but channel your mind to think on the things God tells you.

Letting Go

After you learn to control your thoughts through God's plan for mind renewal by reading His Word, praying and learning to channel your mind to think on His thoughts, another godly process is needed. It is so simple that many people miss it. I call it "letting go." Many of God's people may be able to do all of the things I've mentioned so far, but when it comes to this one, they really have a tough time. They just can't "let go" of their own personal problems.

As I've said earlier, your greatest power is the power of choice. You must choose to think God's way and give up your own thoughts for real peace and contentment. You must continually learn to "let go" of carnal things and opt for spiritual things. If you don't, you'll be reaping the consequences of carnal thinking which is mental and emotional death. "For to be carnally minded is death; but to be spiritually minded is life and peace" (Rom. 8:6). Life in the Spirit is the only way to live. It's restful, it's invigorating, and it's positively life supporting, but you've got to let go of the carnal and opt for the spiritual. You can't live in the Spirit with your own pet problems.

I've traveled around the world on three different occasions. Once, when I was in India, I became fascinated with how they capture monkeys there. They take a jar with an opening just large enough for a monkey's open paw and go into the jungle regions where the monkeys live in the wild. Then they place the jar on the ground, make a trail of nuts leading up to the jar, and finally put some nuts in the jar itself so the monkey can see them. When this is complete, the hunters simply back off and wait. Soon a monkey descends from the trees and starts eating the nuts. He eats his way to the jar. When he sees the nuts inside the jar, he reaches in and grabs the nuts, forming a fist that can't be extracted from the jar. He won't let go of the nuts no matter what; therefore, he becomes trapped. He doesn't have the intelligence to let go of his prize so that he might escape with his life. He holds on even though that large jar on his paw frustrates him to no end. The hunters come out, throw a net over him, and he's caught.

People are like monkeys in that way sometimes. Even when they're emotionally distraught, they won't let go of their prize problems and conflicts no matter what. They can't and won't let go of their problems and difficulties to God or anyone else because they've made up their minds that those are "their" problems and difficulties. Their tenacious, little mental fists cling to their problems, and they become caught in a net of frustration and perplexity.

In London, England, there is a Dr. Bach who has done extensive research into the relationship between emotional illness and physical illness. He claims he can tell his patients' emotional states prior to the onset of their physical diseases. In other words, by analyzing their physical afflictions, Dr. Bach can tell what kind of emotions the patients had *before* they became sick. This shows that different forms of mental and emotional stress cause corresponding physical ailments. It's the stress that does it. Often, I have to tell my patients, "Don't be a monkey, let go!"

I've developed a remarkable theory. It's based upon years of counseling both as a physician and a minister. I believe that most of the nervous disorders I've come across are caused by people trying to boss God, other people, or their circumstances around! I would venture to say, from similar research that I've read, that most of the nervous breakdowns in this country are caused by the same frustrations. You see, people become so frustrated by their inability to do these three things that they eventually go into a tailspin and emotionally collapse. That's why I tell my patients, "Don't be a monkey, let go!" When people see this they are able to analyze most of their problems and help themselves.

I once treated a minister's wife who had suffered a nervous breakdown. Before her breakdown life had become so intolerable for her that she couldn't even go to church to hear her husband preach. She loved and respected him very much. When she did go, she would become so nervous in the presence of all those people that she would flee. I had seen her on several occasions and after a number of visits, I frankly blurted out, "Now, sister, tell me. Who or what are you trying to boss around that won't stay bossed?"

"Well—er—what did you say, Dr. Miller?" she stammered, slightly shocked at the directness of my question. I repeated it. Then she looked at her husband who was with her this day. "Shall we tell him?" she asked him meekly. He nodded with a sigh of relief, and she then continued. "Well, it's like this. My husband's mother is living with us, and she simply won't do what I tell her. Anytime I ask her to do something, she resists me."

"That's the core of your problem. You can't boss her around, right?"

"Yes, but—"

"Listen, you never will be able to," I continued, explaining that the mother-in-law probably had a certain amount of jealousy against her in the first place for taking away her son. This, coupled with the fact that she was getting old, made her less flexible.

"You're not going to change her mind one bit, but you can change yours," I continued. Then I shared with her that instead of trying to boss around her mother-in-law, she should "let go" of the situation and release it to God. This minister's wife had to let go of her frustration and "let" the peace of God flow through her no matter what the circumstances were like at home. It was impossible to boss around her mother-in-law, but she could change her own mind and "let go" of the situation and "let" God have His way in the matter.

Neither the minister nor his wife had ever thought of dealing with the situation like this, but she agreed to give it a try. Well, I saw her the next day and asked how she was feeling. She confided in me that for the first time in months she'd had a good night's sleep! What did she do? She merely "let go." And by so doing—by emotionally "turning the other cheek"—the scriptural truth became perfectly clear to her how she had the choice to "let go" and "let God."

Paul said, "Let the peace of God rule in your hearts" (Col. 3:15). You have to do the "letting." First you have to "let go" and then you have to "let" God's peace rule in your heart. But again, *you* are the center of the decision-making process. Do you know how to "let"? Can you "let go," or are you like the monkey, still clinging to its prize? If you are in the latter category you find yourself caught in a net of frustration and despair.

God gives you a marvelous invitation through Paul's advice to "let go" of your problems and to "let" His peace come into you instead. There's a wealth of spiritual truth and untold peace here if you can receive it. You might feel like you've been running a collision course through life. Even so, you can lean back in the arms of Jesus and believe Him when He says, "Let not your heart be troubled" (John 14:1). Can you let God handle the matter for you? You've seen the price you've been paying by trying to do it for yourself. When you let go and let God's peace rule, nothing contrary to the will of God will be able to invade your life. That's a promise. "When a man's ways please the Lord, he maketh even his enemies to be at peace with him" (Prov. 16:7).

At the Mayo Clinic, where I've visited and studied over the years, they say that about 80 percent of all the people who go there for treatment are depressed, have nervous problems, or are trying to cope with situations they cannot master. The statistics prove that because of their emotional problems, most patients at the Mayo Clinic are treated for physical diseases resulting from emotional frustration. So don't be a monkey; let go!

Believing

Believing is probably the most dynamic factor in the universe. Believing, having faith, expecting something to come into existence that does not already exist make up the grist of the Christian life. Through believing, God has provided not only a way to renew your mind, but also a way in which to alter your circumstances. Books have been written about it, thousands of sermons have been preached on it, but very few people seem to understand the basic rudiments of believing. Jesus said, "If thou canst believe, all things are possible to him that believeth" (Mark 9:23). Just meditate upon that for a moment. It simply means nothing is impossible if you believe.

There are so many principles in God's Word that apply to anyone who believes them. You don't have to be a Bible scholar. You don't have to be a Christian for fifty years. In fact, you don't even have to be a Christian to have many of God's principles work in your life. Whether a saint or sinner applies them, they work; because they are part of God's spiritual laws of the universe. In this sense they are like His physical laws which work for anyone who applies them. The law of gravity applies to anyone who lives on this earth. Likewise, the law of believing applies to anyone who chooses to use it in his life.

I'm sure you know people who have displayed tremendous faith. You've read of accounts of people who have overcome tremendous physical, cultural or financial handicaps by simply believing they could do it. They simply believed and it happened. One time I had a patient who erroneously believed something I did to her was making her well. In reality, it had no medical basis, but just the fact that she believed it did help her get well.

Years ago, while I was practicing in Pennsylvania, I received a call from a Polish immigrant coal miner. In his broken English he conveyed to me that his wife was very sick and I should come immediately. There was a flu epidemic in that area at that time; and sure enough, when I arrived and diagnosed her condition, it was the flu. I left her some medicine—enough for about a week—and told her husband he should call me only in case of an emergency and instructed him how often to give her the medicine—one tablespoon every four hours.

The next day I received a call from the same coal miner telling me his wife was doing much better but that I had better come again—right away. He told me she needed some more medicine. I knew if she had taken all that medicine in one night, she could really be sick, so I hurried out to see them again. When I arrived in their home, I found her sitting up and looking much better than the day before. I picked up the bottle of medicine I had left the night before and noticed that only one or two doses had been taken. I turned to the man and said in a somewhat irritated tone of voice, ''I thought you said she needed more medicine.''

He said, ''She did, but it was not the kind of medicine in the bottle; rather it was the kind you gave to her under her tongue.''

It took me a few moments before I realized what he meant. Both of them thought the thermometer I had placed under her tongue was a form of medication. Just believing that the thermometer was medicine helped her to recover, and she actually got better.

Believing is a function of both your soul (mind) and your spirit. This is very important to understand. It's not just the power of positive thinking, though that plays a part as we shall see; but true believing takes place on both the mental and spiritual planes of your existence. It's when this scriptural believing is merged in both your mind and spirit that things begin to happen.

Salvation is a prime example of this. When you were saved you believed with both your mental and spiritual natures. ''If thou shalt confess with thy mouth [an act of speech stemming from the conscious mind] the Lord Jesus, and shalt believe in thine heart [the inner man of the spirit] that God hath raised him from the dead, thou shalt be saved'' (Rom. 10:9). Salvation isn't just thinking Jesus is Lord. It's thinking it and believing it down in your spirit. When the conscious mind and the spirit work together as one, that's true believing. When you accepted Christ, I trust you had an experience like that. Your mind and your heart were united in faith. You believed.

It is important to remember that true believing utilizes both aspects of your being, and it's believing that will bring anything into existence or alter any circumstance. ''Therefore I say unto you, What things soever ye desire, when ye pray, believe that ye receive them, and ye shall have them'' (Mark 11:24). Jesus said it's not the praying so much as the believing that gets the job done. Believing makes prayer a reality; prayer doesn't make believing a reality. You have to believe first to get results.

The Bible says, "Yea, happy is that people, whose God is the Lord" (Ps. 144:15); and I'm a happy man. I'm seventy-eight years old at the writing of this book and have lived a full and abundant life by the grace of God. I plan to live many more years in the same manner if the Lord should tarry. Now many people say to me, "Don't you know, Dr. Miller, that the Bible says a man's years are three score and ten?" (Ps. 90:10). Then they look at me as though I should all of a sudden accept that, sit down, and give up the ghost.

I believe that when David wrote that he was describing the prevalent condition at his time. He was saying that in his day most men lived a full life at threescore and ten years, but I happen to believe that the normal age was decreed for man in Genesis 6:3, just prior to the flood, when God said, "My spirit shall not always strive with man, for that he also is flesh: yet his days shall be an hundred and twenty years." God allowed Moses to live that long: "And Moses was an hundred and twenty years old when he died: his eye was not dim, nor his natural force abated" (Deut. 34:7). This is what I choose to believe; that is, I accept this with all my heart (spirit) and soul (mind).

When I testify of God's provision in my life, many people think I have an exceptional testimony. That's because I truthfully say I don't know of a single prayer I've ever made for myself or my family that has gone unanswered! God answers prayer. He says, "All things are possible to him that believeth" (Mark 9:23), and I believe that. He says, "What things soever ye desire, when ye pray, believe that ye receive them, and ye shall have them" (Mark 11:24); I believe that too. God has given me the desires of my heart because I've delighted myself in Him and His Word. I don't think there is anything exceptional in my testimony. I think it's just part of the normal Christian life available to anyone who will believe for it.

I've learned to continually believe for things. It's not a once-a-week job with me. There doesn't have to be a crisis situation to motivate me to believe and pray. No, I believe every day of my life for things which are not yet a reality to become a reality in my life. I want to share some of the truths I've learned with you, so that you too may begin to believe continually and thereby renew your mind and alter your circumstances by the power of faith.

Unfortunately, it's hard for a lot of people to be truthful with themselves, and Christians are no exception. It's not that this deception is done intentionally, but many people cover up their true desires and feelings under a religious facade. Let me give you an example of this.

Some time ago there was a teacher of God's Word who was teaching on the topic of believing. He was preaching, "You can have what you want—if you know what you want—as a child of God." He insisted that the problem is that most of God's people don't really know what they want. But he believed that if they ever really discover what the desires of their hearts are, God will fulfill His Word and grant their desires to them.

A sister came up to him after one of his meetings and said, "Brother, the desire of my heart is that my son-in-law would get saved. I've been praying for him for years and nothing ever changes." This minister wisely held to his position, and told her to go home and talk it over with the Lord to see what the problem was. He still maintained, like I do, that God will give us the desires of our hearts.

That night the Lord spoke to this woman. What He said shocked her into reality, but it was true. He told her she couldn't care less whether her son-in-law got saved. He told her she really didn't care two bits whether her son-in-law went to heaven or hell! But what she really wanted was that he would stop abusing her daughter! He treated her daughter very cruelly and this grieved the mother very much. What she wanted—the desire of her heart—was that he would stop mistreating her daughter. The desire of her heart was not his salvation, but she covered over the true desire with a learned, religious platitude. She said she wanted him to get saved, when she just wanted him to stop intimidating her daughter.

Have you ever done that? Have you ever deceived yourself into praying a "religious" prayer, instead of believing for God to grant you the true desire of your heart simply because you are His child? It's crucial that you understand this principle. You must be truthful with yourself and with God. When this woman discovered the phoniness in her prayer, she prayed and believed from her heart that her son-in-law would stop abusing her daughter. Guess what happened—he got saved! And of course after he got saved, he stopped mistreating her daughter. But first the woman had to get truthful with God, before she could really believe. Once she did, God granted her the desire of her heart.

You must be truthful with God. You must be truthful with yourself. If you're financially destitute and need a new car and some new clothes, don't pray for a used car with a hundred thousand miles on it and an old black suit to show off your dandruff. Don't be embarrassed to tell your heavenly Father what you really need and start believing for it.

Kinesiology is a modern study that has shed a tremendous amount of light on the relationship of believing and your subconscious. You see, what you put into your subconscious is what will come out. If you allow negative or untruthful information to permeate into your subconscious spirit, it will definitely affect you in every area of your life. If, on the other hand, you put into your subconscious truthful information and desires, it will determine the type of person you'll become. That's how you'll think, believe and act.

Dr. John Diamond, a personal friend of mine, has specialized in the field of kinesiology in New York for some time. My specialized field of medical study over the years has been that of metabolism and endocrinology. I've been able to substantiate many of Dr. Diamond's findings from my own studies in endocrinology.

Kinesiology demonstrates how anything bad for you, emotionally or physically, will weaken your whole physical body. Conversely, anything that is good for you, emotionally or physically, will strengthen your body. Endocrinology is the branch of medicine dealing with the glands. In your chest, there is a gland called the thymus. This single gland serves as a monitor to your entire nervous and muscular systems. These two systems in turn are part of a much larger system called the "immune system," which consists of all the physiological elements and systems within your body that are designed to protect you from invading disease and keep you healthy. It fights invading bacteria and germs. When your immune system is healthy, so are you. When it is weakened, you are more susceptible to disease.

Your thymus gland is a key organism in triggering your immune system. From this one gland God has marvelously devised a network in your body that tries to protect you from evil, disease and negative emotions. The way it works is that whenever you experience something through your five senses or thoughts, the thymus gland automatically reacts by monitoring your nervous and muscular systems, causing them to be either strengthened or weakened. If you eat something bad for you such as refined sugar, or hear something bad for you such as sad news, or even *think* negatively, or see something bad for you that affects your emotions or moods, your entire physical body will be weakened by the thymus gland which monitors your muscular and nervous systems. You can discover very easily how this works by doing this simple test from the study of kinesiology.

First, cut out some pictures from a magazine. Advertisements often work very well. Some of the pictures should be of pleasant scenes or pleasant-looking faces of people who are happy and content. Then cut out some pictures of people who look depressed, sad or tense. With the help of a friend, do the following: extend your arm perpendicular from your body at a right angle, parallel to the ground, and make a fist. Have your friend apply pressure to your fist by trying to push your arm down. Then resist. Your friend shouldn't try to wrestle you down, but he should simply apply about ten pounds of pressure downward. Normally you will be able to resist.

Then have your friend hold a picture of a pleasant scene or a happy face in front of you and repeat pushing down on your arm. Continue to resist, and as you look at this pleasant picture you will be able to withstand his pressure. Now remove the pleasant picture and replace it with one of sad or depressed faces and look at it. Have your friend exert pressure once more, and you'll find that your arm weakens and gives in quite a bit. Your nervous and muscular systems have weakened as you look at the sad picture.

This is not the result of a thinking process, but the thymus gland is designed to monitor your muscular and nervous systems when anything negative enters through any of your senses. Try it over and over again, and you'll find the same reactions. Sad, depressed, or negative pictures will weaken you, while happy, pleasant pictures will cause you to remain strong.

It has been established that other negative forces, through other senses, work in just the same way. Rock music weakens a person while symphonic or religious music strengthens him. Using the same arm test you can see how sugar or tobacco will cause your arm to weaken. Stretch out your arm again and have your friend try to push it down. You'll be able to resist. Then take a teaspoon of sugar and allow it to melt in your mouth for about thirty seconds and you'll find your arm muscles will weaken if he applies pressure again. For everyone I've ever tested in this manner, the arm became weak; and they could not hold it up against the pressure. With tobacco you don't even have to smoke it or put it in your mouth. Simply look at a cigarette or a cigarette advertisement from a magazine and your arm will automatically weaken under pressure.

The point of this study is to show you that negative forces of any sort will weaken you physically. But since we're dealing with the renewing of your mind, I want to demonstrate how negative thinking and emotions affect you. You've already seen how positive or pleasant pictures affect you when compared to negative or sad ones. Apply this now to your television and movie watching habits, and it will revolutionize your viewing habits. You'll no longer want to allow any debilitative images to enter your mind.

Sometimes I use that arm test on patients, and I say to them, "Imagine you've just received a notice from the Internal Revenue Service saying you owe them $5,000 in back taxes." Guess what? Their arms weaken right away at that bad news, even though it's imaginary. Their thymus gland is still activated by this make-believe bad news. Then I'll say to them, "Imagine your son or daughter has just been graduated from high school with the highest honors!" When they imagine this, their arm remains strong; and they're able to resist my pressure. Good news keeps you strong.

No wonder the Bible tells us to think on those things that are true, honest, just, pure, lovely and of good report. God knows that by channeling your mind to dwell upon such things as these, it will strengthen you. If you think on such things with your conscious mind, it will permeate your subconscious; and you'll begin to believe for greater and better things to happen all the time. But you've got to guard against those negative forces making entry.

I mentioned earlier that I believe it's God's intention for a man to live a full life of one hundred and twenty years. I choose to believe this because of what God's Word says about it. It's not unreasonable to believe what God states as truth. So I don't listen to those who say I should be dead already, but I believe to live for many more fruitful, abundant years.

Here's what I do to augment, or to keep believing for this truth. I have placed around my bathroom medicine cabinet pictures of healthy people who are well over one hundred years old! I choose to let those images enter my mind—images of people who have lived healthy, robust lives.

It is true that I'm around sick people all the time in my practice. I sign many death certificates for people who have died of heart attacks and cancer every year, but in spite of my workaday experiences, I choose to believe and think on those lovely things that are promised to me by the Word of God. I visualize these in my mind continually. Remember what you put into your subconscious through your conscious mind is what will come out. You can believe continually by feeding your subconscious truthful, positive affirmations and visualizations. As you've seen from this brief study of kinesiology and from what the Word proclaims, what you think affects your total health. "And be renewed in the spirit of your mind" (Eph. 4:23).

A good way to find out the condition of your heart is to monitor the way you speak. Start listening to the way you talk about yourself, others and the world. Your speech will indicate the condition of your heart—not your physical heart—but your spirit. "Out of the abundance of the heart, the mouth speaketh" (Matt. 12:34). The things you talk about the most are the things you're thinking about the most and believing for continually.

The world system is based upon fear, doubt and unbelief; in other words, it is based on believing the worst will happen. Millions of people tune in daily to listen to a news broadcast that should be called "bad news." That's what news broadcasts consist of chiefly—bad news (i.e. murders, plane crashes, crime, scandals and so forth). Of course, a percentage of this information is vital to our keeping abreast of things, but the majority of the news is bad news. It's not edifying. A daily diet of that kind of mental preoccupation without anything positive to counter it produces negative people. And negative people, we've discovered, are more prone to become weakened and sick. There's an old expression you've heard, "The early bird catches the worm." I like to remind people who are gruff-spoken and negative that "The surly bird catches the germ!"

Check yourself on this. The news media is always talking about the "unemployment" rate. Now do you parrot the world's negative way of talking about this subject and speak of the 5 percent unemployment rate, or do you talk about the 95 percent employment rate? Most people talk about the small percentage of unemployed and constantly worry about it as a result, but few talk about the exceedingly higher and more positive truth that there are 95 percent of the population out working and trying to better themselves and their families. The fact is there will always be those who don't want to work. There will always be the poor as Jesus said (Matt. 26:11).

However, we're concerned about you—about altering your ways of thinking and believing. Both statements about the employment rate are true. The challenge to you is which way will you view the statistic? Are you going to go with the prevailing, negative world's concern, or are you going to be thankful that so many people are working and emphasize that?

I always teach people to use positive affirmations. I tell them to never say, "I have forgotten." Instead, I encourage them to say, "I have trouble recalling, but it will come to me shortly." When you give a command to your subconscious such as, "I have forgotten," it will follow it out until it receives another command to counter it. You won't be able to remember because you've said to your subconscious, "Don't remember. You have forgotten." You've given yourself a command, "Do not remember." As I've said before, what you put into your subconscious is what will come out. When you tell your subconscious, "It will come to me shortly," you're giving a positive command to your subconscious memory to bring forth the information hidden there. Try this, and you'll be amazed to see the difference it will make in your memory.

Many studies by psychologists and psychiatrists have proven beyond the shadow of a doubt that everything you have ever experienced in your life is not forgotten but stored in your memory bank. Your mind is like a computer in this way. It's loaded with millions of pieces of information on every level. Under the right circumstances and with the right training all of it can be brought forth.

One time I was asked to help a man who had "lost his mind." He was functioning like a vegetable because he had literally refused to accept the reality of his life; so he "lost his mind." However, under truth serum by medical injection this same man was able to tell us how and when this happened and what was the cause for him doing this extremely negative act. He helped us to diagnose his own case. He had all the information stored in his subconscious.

When you say, "I have forgotten," you're actually blocking

the information in your memory bank. Next time you can't recall a person's face, or name or something of that nature, simply say, "I have trouble recalling, but it will come to me shortly." Then continue whatever you are doing and you'll discover that you will remember because you've given your subconscious a command to remember instead of commanding it to forget.

The Bible says, "Thou art snared with the words of thy mouth" (Prov. 6:2). Your words are powerful, more powerful than you have probably realized until now. They not only affect others, but they affect you too! The power of believing is accentuated by the way you speak. The way you speak affects you mentally, emotionally, and physically. Stop snaring yourself with your words. Cultivate the habit of finding the positive aspect of a matter and accentuate it, especially when it applies to your own life. It takes no effort to be negative, because that's the way most people act, talk and think in our society. It's the world's system of fear, doubt and believing for the worst to happen. It's the natural thing that your natural mind wants to do. But you've already discovered that your natural mind is God's worst enemy and that He's provided wonderful ways of renewing it, thereby giving you total health. By speaking right, you're conditioning yourself to believe right.

I want to emphasize again the need to be truthful as you begin to apply the principles of positive affirmations and visualizations to your subconscious. Some people get so excited about this concept once they grasp it that they forget to maintain that truthfulness in the way they phrase things. If you're not truthful, your subconscious mind won't react in accordance with the positive statements that are made. The Bible says that a "double minded" man is not to expect anything from the Lord (James 1:6-8). True believing cannot operate when there is double mindedness, and my definition of double mindedness is a state of mind where there is conflict between your conscious and subconscious mind.

During the 1920s, while I was still a medical student, there was a man by the name of Coue who was from France. He was traveling all over America lecturing people on how to improve their lot in life. He was teaching them that if they would repeat the expression, "Every day in every way, I'm getting better and better," they would improve their health and well-being. You've probably heard or used that expression yourself, as it is almost a cliché today. This sytem of auto-suggestion became extremely popular, but the truth of the matter is that it won't work, and it can be very dangerous.

One of my patients tried to apply this system to his life, and it ended in disaster. He was a physician himself, but he had a very serious heart condition. He told me he was applying Coue's system, and I cautioned him against it for reasons which I'll explain shortly. This doctor actually made a tape recording that went like this, "Every day in every way my heart is getting stronger and stronger." He would go to sleep at night listening to it and wake up in the morning listening to it: "Every day in every way my heart is getting stronger and stronger." However, his subconscious knew that his heart wasn't getting stronger and stronger and could not accept this information. It conflicted with the truth of the matter. One morning they found this doctor dead from a heart attack in his bed with the tape recorder going, "Every day in every way my heart is getting stronger and stronger."

You might say, "What's the difference between Coue's system and yours, Dr. Miller? Aren't you both talking positively and speaking positive affirmations into your subconscious?" Yes, but let me emphasize the need to be truthful. You must never lie to your subconscious. Don't say you're well when you're sick. Don't say you're getting better when you're not. This is presumption rather than belief, and it's lying to your subconscious which knows the truth. This is what this doctor was doing. He was saying he was going to get better when, in fact, he was getting worse every day. He was not acknowledging the sickness and was trying to cover over a truth his subconscious knew. The result was conflict. This was a form of double mindedness. When you're saying you're getting better and better, and it's true you actually are, that's fine. But if you're making this statement and it's not true, your subconscious knows you're lying and won't follow through. You're double minded. If you say you're well when you're sick, your subconscious rebels against it.

It is vital to remember that the subconscious cannot deal in "processes" but only in completed concepts. Your mind thinks in pictures, not processes. To say, "I'm getting better and better," is trying to feed a process to your subconscious. It can't respond to a process but only to a completed concept or picture.

To say a simple phrase like "a normal, healthy body" is feeding a completed concept to your subconscious. "A normal, healthy body" is a phrase that doesn't lie; it expresses the desire of your heart without saying it's in a process of becoming. Your subconscious can accept this because it's a complete concept. You're not saying you have it, yet you're merely expressing the truthful desire of your heart which your subconscious can accept. It's a completed picture, "a normal, healthy body." Your subconscious can visualize this. I never tell people to say they are well when they are sick, but I do tell them to visualize a completed picture by choosing the right words to express the true desire of their hearts. Never try to believe in a process, but begin to believe and visualize the completed concept. Find simple words to express this and repeat them over to yourself daily.

For years I've repeated the expression "a normal, healthy

body" to myself whenever I think about it. This is a true desire of my heart. I even have this and other simple desires written out and placed where I can see them from time to time and repeat them. I've been doing this for years, and I can honestly say that in all of my adult years I've never had a confining illness. That's not to say that I haven't had a few minor maladies, but I believe by expressing that phrase "a normal, healthy body" to my subconscious over these years, I've exempted myself from any confining diseases. This, of course, is in conjunction with observing natural laws of health and diet which we'll talk about in the final section of this book.

If you were in a room full of snakes, it would be sheer foolishness to deny the existence of the snakes. You'd be lying to yourself. The snakes are there, but you don't have to claim them as your own! That's quite different than if you were to deny their existence. Well, the snakes are like a disease. Don't deny its existence, but don't claim it either. I had a woman patient once who was a Christian Scientist, and she came to me quite ill, but said her church didn't believe in sickness. I told her, "Ma'am, you're only perfuming the garbage can. You must admit there's something here that isn't right, but you don't have to identify yourself with it." Speak the truth but separate yourself from things that are negative. Don't deny them but don't identify with them either. Let me give you another true instance to show you what I mean.

I was conducting a series of evangelistic meetings in a church in Alabama once, and we were having prayer for the sick at the end of the service. A lady came forward who had a cancerous growth on her face and said to me, "I've got this cancer and I need prayer." I told her to stop saying, "*I've* got this cancer," because every time she was making this statement, she claimed it as her own. I told her to stop identifying with it. It wasn't her cancer. It wasn't God's cancer. It was of the devil, and she shouldn't lay claim to it in any shape or form. I told her to go home and start speaking that way.

She went home, but the next night she came back in jubilation, for the cancer was no longer on her face! She testified, "I just stopped talking about my cancer. Instead I acknowledged a cancer on my face. It's not mine. It's not from God, and I rebuke it in Jesus' name!" She then reported that the cancer literally fell off her face when she talked that way and was healed. God healed her and the power was in the name of Jesus, but also in the right confession. She stopped claiming the disease as her own.

The point I'm making is that she acknowledged its existence but she separated herself from the entire, negative, satanic thing and spoke the positive word of God! She didn't say she was well when she was sick, but she separated herself from the sickness and refused to accept it as hers. She didn't lie to her subconscious. She wasn't double minded. She spoke the truth without being snared with the words of her mouth. She separated herself from the negative force.

When I was a young man, I used to envision a beautiful house on a beautiful lake with lots of water and swimming fowl. I have such a home today in such a setting, but I'm sure I wouldn't have had it if I didn't picture it, visualize it, speak it and feed it into my subconscious mind continually. I wouldn't have had it, if I didn't believe for it. I would say, "a beautiful house on a beautiful lake" over the years, and now I have it. I didn't say I had it when I didn't, but I expressed in a few words the completed concept of the desires of my heart. I started believing for it by putting pictures of it and speaking of it to my subconscious mind or spirit. I was speaking and seeing it before it came into being. "Now faith is the substance of things hoped for, the evidence of things not seen" (Heb. 11:1). What's the evidence of things not seen? Speaking it, visualizing it, until the unseen evidence becomes seen evidence.

If I say, "I have good eyesight," when I don't, I am lying. But if I visualize it, this is an expression of my heart that my subconscious can accept. The key to really believing in this manner is finding the right word or phrase that presents a truthful, completed concept to your subconscious mind. When you are sick, don't say, "I'm well." Say "good health" or "a normal healthy body" as I do. Keep it simple. Keep it truthful and a completed concept.

The enemy of your soul would like to keep you looking at your limited circumstances and evaluating them with your natural, conscious mind. Instead use your conscious mind to feed your subconscious with positive affirmations and visualizations of the true desires of your heart. God's resources are unlimited. Identify with Him—not the negative forces. Look for the good. Think on the good. Speak the good.

Once I was preaching to a church in Carlsbad, New Mexico, on the subject of the mind and positive affirmations, and after the service a brother in the Lord came up to me and shared this little poem that he had picked up some place.

> If you talk about your troubles
> And tell them o'er and o'er
> Then the world will think you like them
> And proceed to give you more.

5

BALANCING YOUR EMOTIONS

Not only does God set you free from the tyranny of your natural mind by giving you authority over it as we've just discussed, but He has provided a balanced way of living for His people so they could let their light shine in the midst of a hectic and confused generation. God is the author of balance in His creation and in your life. In Ecclesiastes 3, we read of His care in balancing life and nature, "To every thing there is a season, and a time to every purpose."

God doesn't expect you to do more than you're capable of performing. He doesn't expect you to be other than what He created you to be from the beginning. This is so clearly evidenced in the parable of the talents in Matthew 25:14-30. The Lord gives to each one of us talents "according to his several ability." What He gives to us, He expects us to use. You and I are not expected to move the whole world. We have a purpose to fulfill, a job to do, designed by the Master Potter, just as the man with the one talent in the parable. This man was expected to do something with his talent, but he wasn't expected to do the work of the person with two talents or the person with five talents.

God has made provision for us to live abundant, balanced

lives for Him within the scope of the abilities and desires He has planted in us. If Paul could say, "But by the grace of God I am what I am" (1 Cor. 15:10), so can you. Believe for great things. Think on good things. Speak positive words of life to yourself and others, but don't try to be more than what God has made you to be.

I've lived an active, fulfilling life with my wife, Elizabeth. We've raised four wonderful children. I've been blessed with a professional life that has allowed me to care for congressmen and cabinet members. I've been invited to two presidential inaugurations. In addition to these honors, I've had my own radio program, conducted evangelistic meetings, served as a dean of a Bible school, pioneered five different churches, edited several publications, and directed a large medical clinic in addition to my own prospering medical practice. Life has been full and busy.

All this has required me to learn how to balance my life and my emotions. A book I read in medical school has helped me to do that. It is entitled *What Men Live By*, by Dr. Richard Cabot, who was professor of medicine and social ethics at Harvard University. The book has been out of print for some time, but if you can dig up a copy somewhere, I suggest that you read it. Dr. Cabot diagnosed man's emotional needs into four basic categories which he termed work, play, love and worship. He goes into extensive detail in subdividing these categories, but I have found that by keeping it simple and changing the word "worship" to "God" I have been able to help a lot of people balance their lives emotionally.

Using these four categories, I have also developed my own diagram that has been helpful when I've been lecturing on this subject. I'll usually draw a small circle in the middle of the blackboard with four equal lines stemming out from the perimeter of the circle forming a cross. Each stem of the cross is equidistant from the circle or hub at the center. Imagine, if you will, the hub of a wheel with four spokes coming out, forming a cross. At the top of the cross I put the word "God." At the bottom, "love." At the left side, "work." At the right side, "play." These represent the four basic facets of man's emotional life. All four of these must be equally exercised and kept in the same proportion to each other for a person to enjoy an emotionally balanced, happy life.

The hub of the wheel turns depending on the pace of life you choose to live. The pace of life which you live can be either slow or fast. It's not the pace of life that harms you, but what really destroys you is the wheel being out of balance as it turns. The wheel goes out of balance if one of the four spokes, or four sections of the cross, grow out of proportion to the rest. If one segment of the cross is longer than another, it will throw the whole wheel out of balance as the hub of your life spins. So, the more nearly you keep the four segments balanced, the better off you're going to be. All four must be equally balanced—God, love, work and play.

An automobile mechanic once told me that a car wheel with only a seven-ounce imbalance will produce thirteen pounds of imbalance on that wheel when it's spinning at fifty miles per hour. That's like thirteen pounds of pressure on that tire at that speed, and it will eventually ruin the ride. This is a good example of what happens to you when your life is not in balance according to these four needs. The faster you go, the more stress you will feel. The bumps of life will take their toll at an earlier age.

If you do not accept the power of God in your life, then you will not be a balanced person. This is at the top of the cross diagram. You need to depend on the Lord who is greater than you. You need His divine help to cope with life. You must recognize Him as the Lord of your life.

At the bottom of the cross there is the word "love." There must be a place to dwell where there is love, warmth and peace—a place where these feelings and emotions can be expressed. Ideally, it's the home. It doesn't mean you have to be married, but it does mean you have a place to live where everything is congenial. In this place there is love, fellowship and friendship. This segment of the cross must be the same length as the godward one.

There are many ministers today who work for God. They do a great deal for God, but they spend too little time with their families. The result is often disastrous as in the case of one preacher I knew who I'll discuss in a while. I often think of this Scripture as reflecting balance: "And Jesus increased in wisdom and stature, and in favour with God and man" (Luke 2:52).

The left side of the cross represents the "work" area of man's life. This is what you do that has to be done in order to earn a living and to fulfill your obligations. Hard work never hurt anyone. Remember it's the stress of leading an unbalanced life that destroys—not hard work (barring any physical limitations). The person who works hard must play hard! This is a key of balance on the right side of the cross.

"Play" is doing something you want to do that does not have to be done. As soon as it has to be done, it becomes work and is no longer play. God, love, work and play—these are the four facets of your life that have to be kept in balance at all times to live a healthy, happy life.

The minister mentioned earlier was a patient of mine who literally worked himself to death. Again, it wasn't the hard work, but it was the stress from not balancing his hard work with the other aspects of his needs that caused the problem. This is the cause for so much hypertension today. He had very high blood pressure, and I cautioned him to slow down and "play" a little to get him to relax a bit. He emphasized God and work but he grossly neglected the areas of play and love. The pressure built as his pace of life increased. I told him, "Listen, brother, your blood pressure is 220 over 120, and you're going to have to play more, enjoy your family more, and relax—or you're not going to live!"

He answered emphatically, "What? There's so much to be done, I just can't help it. I've got to work! I've got to work!"

Two weeks later he died. Somebody else is now doing his work. None of us is indispensible!

So many of the people I examine are under stress and strain all the time. It's pathetic. If you're a hard worker, you must take time to play. Some of my patients seem dumbfounded by this advice. They ask, "How shall I play? I'm not a kid any more." All playing is doing something you don't have to do. You don't have to play childish games in order to play. It just has to be something you enjoy that doesn't have to be done. It can be raising flowers or painting. It can be doing jigsaw puzzles or bowling. It doesn't matter what type of fun it is, but you must learn to play. It's important to your health. Often when I'm working very hard, it becomes evident to my office staff. Usually one of them will remind me, "Dr. Miller, it's time for you to take a little time off and play again," and I do. I like to travel. I'll get away and take a trip for pleasure. That's play for me. It wouldn't be for a traveling salesman perhaps, but for me it's play.

Now a person who is overbalanced in the play area is what our society has mistakenly glorified as a playboy. And he is the most miserable of creatures. He is always avoiding work. Usually he has no need for God. For if he did, he would find that a playboy's life wouldn't be compatible with God's Word. If he's got the means and the money, he plays golf in the summer, goes skiing in the winter with perhaps yachting or polo in between. He plays with people too, causing havoc with those he gets involved with. Though his outward appearance might sport a handsome tan and a good physique, inwardly he will never be happy or satisfied.

You must balance your emotional needs. That's the way you were created. God doesn't want you to be more than you are, but He has ingeniously made you so that you can live a balanced life for His glory. Using the diagram I've described, diagnose your own problems. Draw a hub in the center of a cross. Are each of the segments of the cross equal in your life? Do they balance out, or are there some glaring imbalances? Are God, love, work and play equally balanced? If you haven't been spending enough time godward, do so. If you see from your personal diagram that you're coming up short at the love end of the cross, start to spend more time at home with your family and loved ones. In my counseling I've met so many people who expressed the regret that they hadn't taken the time to show their love to their family and friends. How they wished they could have spent more time with certain loved ones, but didn't take the time to do it. They didn't choose to make the time, and now it's too late!

I love God, and I've served Him all my life. I'm a professional man with tremendous demands upon my time. I preach, I teach, I work and I play; but I also make sure I spend time with my wife. Elizabeth and I have been happily married for over fifty-five years, and we both find we need each other more the older we get in life. I keep my godward needs balanced with my love needs. I keep my work needs balanced with my play needs. Believe me, this system of balancing your emotional needs works.

If you're one of those hard-working individuals who is constantly under stress and strain, it will show on this diagram. Be honest with yourself. You can't afford not to be. You must find some type of enjoyable play to counter your working pressure.

I like what Jesus said to His disciples who were hard-working men, "Except ye be converted, and become as little children, ye shall not enter into the kingdom of heaven" (Matt. 18:3). Can you imagine Him talking to His followers that way? Can you imagine grown men trying to figure out how to become like children? After they were converted? Study young children and see what they're like. Yes, it's true that they believe very easily which the Lord wants us to do, but another obvious quality of children is that they can enjoy the present moment at the drop of a hat. They love to play and usually find no difficulty in doing this. They don't fret about tomorrow. They don't think about the past, but they're able to get involved in the present. Well, I believe the Lord wants some of us mature, hard-working people to learn to do that too.

Finally, if your life is too occupied with play or pleasures, you need to balance it with work. Aside from the playboy type, I've found that a lot of our senior citizens have been guilty of this malady. They have fallen for the gilded notion that retirement means sitting back and doing nothing but the things they've wanted to do all their lives. This is such a false conception. For me "retire" means to go to bed and stay there until you have to get up. I don't even like to use the word. We have forced a good many people in our nation into compulsory retirement who had a good many more years to creatively produce on their jobs. Others retire on their own, thinking they can just stop work, and begin to leisurely play at things in their latter years. Well, it just doesn't work that way. God intended us to work. Now that doesn't mean you have to do strenuous work when you're older, but it's important to be committed to some form of work if you are physically able.

I live in an area of the country where there are many retired people. I've seen what happens to many of our senior citizens who move down here with a false concept of retiring for the rest of their lives. Too often the results are tragic because these retirees try to eliminate work from their lives completely, and their emotions cannot cope with it.

In 1972 my office caught fire and burned down. It was a complete loss. Many people came to me and said this was a wonderful opportunity for me to close my doors, get out of my profession and retire.

"Listen, dad, you've worked hard enough. Right now is a good time for you to quit. You might just as well collect your insurance and stop worrying," my son told me. He meant well, as did the others who offered the same type of advice. But I was thankful there were others who expressed the desire that I shouldn't quit. I didn't feel I was indispensible, but I felt I was serving a purpose and still had a good many years left to work. So I decided to start all over again, and I did. Out of the ruins of that fire I started a new office at the age of seventy-two, and I have never regretted it.

Remember, it's not the speed at which you live your life, but it's the stress under which you live that causes trouble. If you keep your life in balance (just as the wheels of a car have to be kept in balance to turn smoothly) you can live a productive, happy life in harmony with God and man. So put God first, put love next, put work and play on opposite sides of the hub of your life and then go as fast as you want to. It will spin just as fast as you move according to the talents and abilities which God has given you. As long as you keep your life in perfect balance, you're going to get along just fine. I'd like to close this chapter with a wonderful statement of life by an unknown author:

PROMISE YOURSELF

To be so strong that nothing can disturb your peace of mind.

To talk health, happiness and prosperity to every person you meet.

To make all your friends feel there is something good in them.

To look on the sunny side of everything and try to make your opinion come true.

To think only of the best; work only for the best, and to expect only the best.

To be just as enthusiastic for the success of others as you are for your own.

To forget the mistakes of the past and press on to greater achievement in the future.

To have a cheerful countenance at all times and a smile ready for every living creature you meet.

To give so much time to self-government that you will not have time to criticize others.

To be too big for worry; too noble for malice; too strong for fear, and too happy to permit the presence of trouble.

6

YOUR BODY IS THE TEMPLE

Daniel prophesied about the last days, "Many shall run to and fro, and knowledge shall be increased" (Dan. 12:4). He wasn't just talking about spiritual knowledge, but knowledge in every field of endeavor. I don't think there's a clearer indication that we are in those last days than by the vast amount of knowledge man has accumulated in recent years. It's astounding, and there's no comparable period in history that has seen such a knowledge breakthrough as we have experienced in our day and age.

Our children are growing up in an age when space travel and heart transplants are common topics of conversation. These things were not even thought possible a couple of generations back. I remember the time as a young doctor when I looked down the throat of a child who died a half-hour later of diphtheria, knowing at the time that I was totally helpless in trying to cure her. Yet today childhood diseases like diphtheria, smallpox and polio are, for all ostensible purposes, unheard of in our country because of the medical knowledge that has come about in these last years.

God doesn't want His people kept in ignorance—either spiritually or physically. "What? know ye not that your body is the temple of the Holy Ghost which is in you, which ye have of God, and ye are not your own? For ye are bought with a price: therefore glorify God in your body, and in your spirit, which are God's'' (1 Cor. 6:19, 20). You are to glorify God *in your body* and your spirit. Your body is important to the Lord. He made it. Like your natural mind, your body is to be brought under subjection to and ruled by your spirit (1 Cor. 9:27), but it is still important to God and should be taken care of and treated well. We all know that it's very hard to be spiritual when our bodies are racked with pain or sickness and weakened with disease. It's been my contention for years that much of the physical suffering God's people experience could be corrected or completely eliminated by proper nutritional standards and observance of "natural laws" God has ordained for our benefit.

Inasmuch as we live on a planet from which our bodies are made, there is overwhelming evidence that God has ordained rules and "natural laws" to regulate our bodies and keep them in good health. Yes, I believe certain physical conditions are the result of spiritual problems that only prayer can solve, but at the same time there are certain rules that have to be observed for the body to function properly. In many ways, I can liken our bodies to an automobile.

Just the other day I was driving my car and it started to give me trouble. The engine started "acting up," as I like to say. Well, this was an emergency situation, and I desperately needed my car. Without thinking about it, I quickly prayed, took the authority and rebuked that disturbance in my car's engine in the name of Jesus! And the Lord gave me the power to get to my journey's end without any further trouble. But the next day I took my car into a garage to get it fixed. I don't expect my car to work on prayer continuously. It has to be kept up to function properly. That's the way it's made. If my car runs low on gas, I don't say, "Lord, you fill it." God won't do for us what we can do for ourselves. Your body is made to be operated by food. It's made out of food or nutrients and must be replenished—just as the Lord made so clear when he raised the young girl from the dead in Mark 5:39-43. The last thing He said to the people after He had brought the girl back to life was "something should be given her to eat." He didn't expect this resurrected girl to live on prayer. No, after the miracle was performed, He commanded them to get her some food so she might have some proper nutrition to keep her body going!

In nearly every case where the word "sin" is used in the New Testament, the literal Greek translation for that word means "to miss the mark." That's what sin is, missing the mark, not hitting right on target. Usually, when we think of sin, we think of moral sins. These are certainly important, but I believe there are certain cases where we "miss the mark", and it's not necessarily moral sin. When Jesus healed the impotent man at the pool of Bethesda, He said to him, "Behold thou art made whole: sin no more, lest a worse thing come unto thee" (John 5:1-16). Could He not be saying here, "Don't do the same things that caused you to have this trouble in the first place"? I think it's quite possible. This is why I believe if we do sin against our bodies, God doesn't want us to just be forgiven and do the same thing over and over again. He doesn't want us to continue to miss the mark. People often sin against their bodies with their knives and forks. They don't feed their bodies the proper food. Many people do this when they know it's bad for them. I stand with James on this and say, "Therefore to him that knoweth to do good, and doeth it not, to him it is sin" (James 4:17). Poor nutrition is not a moral sin, but it is missing the mark concerning the physical body. Many other people sin against their bodies just because they don't know any better.

As a physician and a practitioner of naturopathy, God has given me a lifetime of medical research and knowledge that has practically helped thousands of people to keep their "temples" healthy, wholesome places for the Holy Spirit to live. I know the Bible teaches that "the kingdom of God is not meat and drink" (Rom. 14:17); and Jesus made it very clear that "not that which goeth into the mouth defileth a man" (Matt. 15:11). However, here we're not referring to the spiritual truths of kingdom living now. We're talking about that "temple," your body, which houses God's Spirit. You have to take care of your body so it can perform efficiently. It's been proven that people who take care of their bodies lead longer, healthier and happier lives. And this is how you "glorify God in your body."

7

SOMETHING WILL ALWAYS
FILL A VOID, EVEN
IF IT IS ERROR

It's a sad truth that for years there has been a tremendous lack of knowledge among the medical profession about nutritional inadequacies and their relationships to disease. I recently had a brother who spent some time in the hospital for heart surgery. When he came out, I asked him what the surgeon had told him about eating. He said, "Nothing at all."

I said, "You mean to tell me he didn't advise you to avoid the use of refined sugar and flour or salt?"

"Well," my brother thought for a moment, "the doctor said I shouldn't put too much salt on my food." That was the entire extent of nutritional information the doctor had given a man who had just experienced heart surgery. This doctor was a noted surgeon too, but his knowledge of proper nutrition was grossly lacking. He even said that if my brother's food was prepared with salt it would be okay, just not to add too much salt when it's served to him.

I was shocked to hear this, but then on the other hand I realized that most physicians who graduate from medical schools today very seldom, if ever, get any instruction in dietetics. It was the same in my medical studies years ago. When I was a medical student, I learned how to practice medicine on dead bodies and sick people—that's basically the same way it is today.

I have a young, professional acquaintance, a doctor who recently graduated from the University of Alabama Medical School. He told me the only information they received on nutrition in their entire curriculum was a single course of study in which the textbook was published by one of our larger food companies. In actuality the text proved to be not much more than an advertisement for the products which this company manufactured! Most other medical schools today are the same.

Fortunately, during my medical training I was privileged to hear a noted physician, Dr. Eugene Christian, who had cured himself of what was diagnosed as an incurable disease by using food as medicine. He published a series of booklets which I still retain. This gave me my start in using nutrition as a form of medicine too. Dr. Christian discovered that the medicine he had been taking didn't do the job for him that proper nutrition did. He didn't ignore the use of medicine, and neither do I, but we need to remember that there are many conditions we can help by proper diet.

Today, most of our drugs are made from herbs, plants and their derivatives, things which draw their nourishment from the earth; but we forget sometimes that our bodies are made from the dust of the earth too. This is another way of saying that the chemicals in the earth are converted into plant life; we eat these fruits and vegetables, or the animals that eat other plants, and receive our nourishment. Any way you look at it, it all comes out of the earth of which we are made. Now the question is, if we can get some of these substances to help us in the form of drugs or medicines, cannot we also get these substances through proper diet and food, since both are made from the chemicals and nutrients of the earth? The answer is definitely yes!

Recently it was reported that a man at an Eastern university cured an ulcer by eating a large amount of cabbage. They kept asking him why he ate so much cabbage, but he just said it made him feel better. So he continued to eat the cabbage, and his ulcer got better. Today there is a remedy being produced by one of our drug companies that is primarily made from cabbage and it's being used in the treatment of ulcers. This is my point, and something I've put a lifetime of research into, that often men will try all kinds of things to heal a condition rather than just utilizing the wholesome food of the earth God has made for healing diseases. I believe we could avoid many such conditions if we would only adhere more closely to nature.

Now because there has been a tremendous lack of information on proper nutrition within the medical profession and its relationship to health, the result has been a tremendous void in this field. Whenever there is a void in knowledge, something will come along to fill it, even if it's error. And that's what's happened in America within the last generation.

People have become aware of the tremendous inadequacies in their diets caused by much of our modern food processing methods, but they have been floundering for any solid, practical knowledge to fill that void and meet this urgent need. As a result, the entire field of health and food has been flooded by a host of self-proclaimed "experts." Many of these have helped; but many more have hurt the general public, because they didn't have the proper physiological training to understand the complete functioning of the body. Partial truths are also partial falsehoods. And for years health food books have been dominated by people who have been faddists, vegetarians, or involved in the occult. They tie up their dietary regulations with some form of false worship or philosophy. Today when you walk into a health food store, you're more than likely to be confronted by a rack full of books ranging from macrobiotic diets to disciplines in Yoga, all purporting to improve your health through their traditions and advice. It's a sad state, and many people have been trapped into following occult practices through concern for their own physical health. They've realized there must be alternative nutritive methods than those offered to us by our giant food conglomerates which flout them to us continuously via radio, television, newspapers and magazines. People have come to realize more and more that those processed, refined package goodies may appeal to our eyes and taste, but in reality don't have any healthful benefits at all. More often, they're dangerous to our health.

But in their search for a valid dietary program, many of these people have been enslaved to follow all sorts of dietary regimens that are tied into false religious and philosophical systems. For example, vegetarian diets that come from India are based upon the Hindu concept of the transmigration of souls. At death they believe the soul goes from one body into another. They literally don't eat meat, because they feel they may be eating someone's ancestor! Not all vegetarians believe this today, but this is how the basic belief system developed that motivates such a dietary discipline. There are many other fad diets today that stem from similarly erroneous doctrines.

I would wholeheartedly agree that to eat a lot of raw vegetables, or a diet primarily of vegetables for several days or a week at a time is a good thing to do. That's fine. Such a diet has a very good purging effect on your intestines and helps purify anything toxic in your system. But to become a total vegetarian and eliminate protein sources from animal matter is very unwise. Very often vegetarians will tell you Genesis says that God told man to eat only herbs and fruit. This is very true. But it's also true that after the flood God told Noah that he could eat most anything, including the flesh of animals: "Every moving thing that liveth shall be meat for you; even as the green herb have I given you all things" (Gen. 9:3)! Vegetarians won't quote that Scripture, but it was God's command, and as we know, man obeyed it. Some people can get along without meat. Others can't.

When people come to me for aid, I usually give them a series of extensive tests, including a blood test, to measure possible deficiencies. In all my years of practice, while measuring the protein levels of thousands of patients, I have never examined one vegetarian that was not "protein deficient." Some people can get along without meat; nonetheless, they remain somewhat deficient in protein.

Your body is made of protein. You must have protein in order to replenish, repair and rebuild your body as it is worn down by the activities of the day. When a person dies a natural death, one of the usual reasons is that the protein level in the blood has been depleted. So, you must have protein. Proteins are organic compounds made up of amino acids found in a variety of foods. Nuts and beans are good protein foods, but primary protein sources are foods such as meat, fish, seafood, poultry, cheese, milk, yogurt, and eggs. Your body needs protein from all of these sources to constantly replace and repair body tissue.

The purpose of this section of the book is not to suggest that you drastically change your life style or to get you so spend more money on the food you eat, but to teach you to be selective in what and how you eat. This is of the utmost importance. I have pioneered a system of eating that has helped to cure many people over the years who had previously been suffering from intestinal disorders ranging from indigestion to gastric ulcers.

A basic premise that you'll find as a guideline throughout this section is that *if God made it, and man hasn't tampered with it, it's okay for you to eat.* As you read and learn to take care of your body by the observations and methods I have found to be healthful, you might feel at first that the road is too "straight and narrow." And it is. As with your spiritual walk with the Lord, this straight and narrow road will lead to a healthier and happier life too. You won't pray over your food any more like the brother who said, "O Lord, bless what you can on this table, and forgive us for the rest, Amen!" You'll know better.

Physically speaking, you are what you eat, drink, breathe and think. We've already seen this demonstrated rather dramatically from the studies in kinesiology in the last chapter. Anything that enters your body through the senses weakens your nervous and muscular system through that monitoring gland we discovered called the thymus.

The Lord has built into us this automatic, defensive warning system. The fact is there are enough germs in your body at any given time that could kill you if it were not for the fantastic immune system that is greater than the invading bacteria. Basically, physical health consists in keeping your immune system strong enough to resist infection. By discovering the "natural laws" God has provided for His children and applying them to our lives, we can greatly strengthen our immune systems and live in good health.

8

GOD'S NATURAL LAWS ABOUND THROUGHOUT HIS CREATION

The Lord has woven into His universe natural laws which regulate and control what He has created. He is a God of design and precision and not a God of circumstance. From the establishment of the natural forces of the seas to the orbital precision of the galaxies, God has ordained order and regulations. "Or who shut up the seas with doors, And said, Hitherto shalt thou come, but no further: and here shall thy proud waves be stayed?" (Job 38:8, 11). The Lord established the earth and the seas and the skies.

David marveled at the order of the skies as he mused upon the way God had ordained regularity in the heavens. "When I consider the heavens, the work of thy fingers, the moon and the stars, which thou hast ordained; What is man, that thou art mindful of him?" (Ps. 8:3, 4).

It is because God has made himself so obvious to mankind through these natural phenomena of order and precision that He says man is without excuse for refusing to acknowledge Him. "For what can be known about God is plain to them, because God has shown it to them. Ever since the creation of the world his invisible nature, namely, his eternal power and deity, has been clearly perceived in the things that have been made. So they are without excuse'' (Rom. 1:19, 20 RSV). Man can see God in the order and wonder of His universe, a universe regulated by His natural laws.

The law of gravity works for mankind universally. It works in this country. It works in other countries. There is a natural law of gravity that cannot be broken. You can't just say, ''Well, I'm a child of God, and He'll take care of me,'' and then try to walk off a roof or a cliff. That would be near suicide, because God has ordained the law of gravity. It's a law of nature, as we say. If we don't observe it, we suffer the consequences. There is a natural law of locomotion which is simplified in the premise that if I step out in front of a moving object, such as a speeding automobile, I will be killed because I did not observe the law of locomotion. When we try to break the natural laws of God, we never really break them; we only break ourselves upon them.

When I was pastoring a church and practicing as a physician in Washington, D.C., I was invited to speak at a church convention in another region. One of our young people had just bought a new car and was eager to show it off. ''When you go to the convention,'' he said, ''let me drive you. I want you to see how this new car performs.'' I took him up on his offer and went with him.

As we were driving between Washington and Baltimore, he started to speed up quite a bit. I warned him that there was much heavy traffic and that the speed laws were rigidly enforced. He didn't pay much attention to my warnings, because he was so eager to show me what this car could do. It wasn't very long before we heard a siren, and a police car pulled us to the side of the road. The driver was arrested and taken to the constable's office. Since I had a driver's license, I was allowed to take the car and proceed to my destination, but he had to stay in jail because he was fined eighty-five dollars—more money than all of us had put together. After the convention, we all went home and gathered up the necessary cash to bail him out, but it wasn't until well after midnight that he was able to taste freedom again. He was very much chagrined, and I remember he was still shaking when we went to free him.

"I guess I broke the law," he said to me.

"No, William, you didn't break the law. The law is still good and in effect. You have broken yourself upon this law by violating it."

This is what we do when we try to break God's natural laws. We never break them; we only break ourselves upon them and pay the consequences for violating them. This is particularly true when we don't observe God's natural laws of health. We destroy our bodies by ignoring them. I'm speaking specifically of what I term the laws of sanitation, activity and nutrition. I am not implying that we should adhere to the Mosaic dietary laws decreed for the children of Israel under the Old Covenant or the Old Testament. I want to make that very clear.

The Bible makes it clear that the Mosaic Law, which contained dietary laws, was delivered specifically to Israel. "These are the statutes and judgments and laws, which the Lord made between him and *the children of Israel* in mount Sinai by the hand of Moses" (Lev. 26:46).

In the New Testament we find Paul, an apostle to the Gentiles, referring to his kinsmen according to the flesh—Jews, "Who are Israelites; to whom pertaineth the adoption, and the glory, and the covenants, and *the giving of the law,* and the service of God, and the promises" (Rom. 9:4). In Romans 2:14, he again contrasts the Jews who received the law with the Gentiles who did not. This is why Peter, also a Jew, initially protested when the Lord gave him a vision and told him that he had made all food clean to eat (Acts 10:9-16).

The whole debate about Christians keeping the law was finally resolved when the elders of the church established once and for all that they would not try to require the believers in the Messiah to keep the Mosaic Law. It's recorded that they would lay no greater burden upon the believers than to "abstain from meats offered to idols, and from blood, and from things strangled, and from fornication" (Acts 15:29). Make no mistake about it, the "law was our schoolmaster to bring us unto Christ, that we might be justified by faith. But after that faith is come, we are no longer under a schoolmaster" (Gal. 3:24, 25). The entrance of a New Covenant, by faith in Jesus Christ, has set us free from the Law and any type of dietary legalism. In fact the New Testament warns believers about those who would come into the church and try to establish dietary laws. It warns of such brethren who will be "giving heed to seducing spirits, and doctrines of devils . . . commanding to abstain from meats which God hath created" (1 Tim. 4:1-3).

There is no need to bring any person under any type of dietary bondage. What you eat will not make you any more spiritual, it will only make you healthier. That's my purpose. That's my intention. As we study these natural laws of health, laws of sanitation, activity and nutrition, remember: *if God made it, and man hasn't tampered with it, it's okay for you to eat.*

9

LAWS OF SANITATION

"Cleanliness is next to godliness" may not be exactly
scriptural, but it certainly is based upon a scriptural truth.
We've been talking about the Law of Moses and although it
contained dietary provisions, it was much more than that. The
Law was delivered as a complete unit of 613 commandments;
365 are negative and 248 are positive. It covered every area of
life for the people of Israel and was a means of separating them
from the nations around them. There were ordinances for
cleanliness, dealing not only with food preparation, but with
diseased persons, menstruating women, dead bodies and
various ritualistic washings and ceremonies for religious
service. In Deuteronomy 23:13 and 14, we find that God
sanitizes the camp by having the people bury their excrement!
God has commanded His people to be clean. Is it any wonder
that Peter exclaimed, "I have never eaten any thing that is
common or unclean" (Acts 10:14, 15), when God gave him a
vision and a new revelation that all things from now on were
clean?

Very often today, when a person is born again by receiving
Christ as his Savior, he cleans up his way of living. Many
people, as they become new creations in Christ, give up

smoking, alcohol or other habits that are unclean for their bodies. I heard the story of one young couple who experienced salvation together. They were members of the hippie culture and were living in a very filthy house. They didn't have a Bible at first and they weren't going to church, but they knew they had met God. They decided they should pray. The wife remembered the Lord's Prayer from her childhood days in church, and they got down on their knees in their living room and prayed this model prayer. As soon as they were finished, they got up and felt a mutual urge to clean up the living room. They did so. Then they went to the bedroom and got down on their knees and prayed the same prayer. They were moved to clean up that room. And so it went throughout the house, until the entire dwelling was cleaned from the mess it had become as a result of their life style.

I believe the reason for this is that when many people's spirits are born again by the Holy Spirit, they are literally delivered from "unclean spirits," (Mark 5:8; Luke 4:33). When people have a real confrontation with God, they "clean up their act."

God, in the same way, has ordained "natural laws" for cleansing within your physical body. Your body is so constructed that it has built-in natural cleansing systems. If we abuse them, it will cause suffering and ill health.

Your skin is the greatest organ of cleansing and elimination you have. There is continuous emission of waste materials through your skin to the outside air. This is a primary reason for keeping your skin clean. It doesn't mean you should use strong soaps or detergents to keep your skin clean, but regular bathing and washing is important. Keeping your skin clean allows the pores to eliminate waste products as they surface.

Your lungs are probably the next most obvious organs of elimination and cleansing. They take in oxygen and liberate, or release, carbonic acid gas. If you'd like to see how potent the carbonic acid gas that comes from your lungs is, take an old-fashioned kerosene lamp or candle, and cup your hands around its light. Take a deep breath and then slowly exhale on top of the flame. Don't blow hard. Just slowly exhale directly over the flame and you'll see what will happen. The carbonic acid gas in your breath will put out the flame. The carbonic acid gas generated in your body and exhaled through the cleansing mechanism of your lungs is enough to poison the air and put out the flame! Therefore, it's very important to keep the air passages of your lungs open so that you can eliminate poisonous wastes.

I remember when I was a young doctor in Washington, D.C. I observed the coloring of a patient's lungs was usually dark blue. When I moved my practice to Sarasota, Florida, I noticed a difference. The coloring of the lungs in most people there would be light blue. I was naive enough at the time to ask about the difference in lung coloring and found it was due to the lack of air pollution in the South. The pollution and air contaminants in an industrialized area will make the lungs a darker blue. The lungs literally become coated with pollutants. The air pollution problem today is of such a vast magnitude that there are very few places in the nation where one can safely assume he's breathing pure air. Nowadays, it's really a question of degrees of air pollution.

Emphysema is becoming a very prominent disease today. It is thought that most of the time it comes from the use of tobacco, but that's not always the case. There are other things we breathe that will definitely interfere with the proper functioning of the lungs, as in the case of my sister-in-law. She never smoked a cigarette in her life, and yet she is dying of emphysema. I don't mean she is bedridden. The medication we have been able to give her helps her lungs keep open, but I have seen her suffer coughing spasms that make it seem as if she is dying. She has been examined by several doctors. They invariably ask her how long she has smoked and how much she smokes. When she tells them she has never smoked, they are usually quite surprised.

The truth is that many years ago, while she lived in Pennsylvania, her husband had a small farm on which he raised tobacco for a cash crop. He never smoked it or used it himself. Neither did she. One year, my sister-in-law, who is a registered nurse, helped him "strip" the tobacco because they were short of help. This involves taking hold of the tobacco leaves and stripping them off the stem by hand. She did this for only one season, then she developed emphysema. She absorbed that tobacco through her skin just as surely as if she had inhaled cigarette smoke. As a result, her lungs are partially paralyzed. That's what emphysema does.

For several years I was the editor of the *American Journal for Medico-Physical Research* which is published in Chicago. In that position I had access to many government papers and other forms of information that seldom reach the press. In one of these governmental reports I discovered that farmers were using a certain type of insecticide called Deldrin on their tobacco. This literally poisons the tobacco plant. If a person were to inhale the smoke of tobacco on which Deldrin had been used, it would be exactly like inhaling Deldrin itself.

The government issued warnings to the manufacturers of tobacco products that they should not use Deldrin. Tobacco manufacturers already had warehouses full of tobacco with this poison on it—approximately seven years worth of tobacco. They were allowed to manufacture tobacco products from the treated tobacco for seven years until the warehouses were depleted. Cranberries from New Jersey, on the other hand, which had sixty times less Deldrin were destroyed, because they were deemed not fit for human consumption. Nonetheless, the tobacco was allowed to remain on the market!

I believe this is one of the reasons why emphysema is in near epidemic proportions today. The tobacco itself is bad enough for a person's lungs, but very often the insecticides used on it are the cause for emphysema. It's a terrible condition. A person who dies of emphysema smothers to death. I know of one case where a person literally drowned from the secretions in his lungs because they couldn't be expelled in the proper manner.

If you smoke or use tobacco in any form, you should stop. It's imperative that you do so. We've seen, as in the case of my sister-in-law, that you don't have to be a user of tobacco to contract some of its negative effects. When you inhale the tobacco smoke of others you become contaminated just as much as they are. Your lungs are very important organs of elimination and you must keep them clean and open to enable you to enjoy good health. I know there are many Christians who still have the habit of smoking, but the Lord is faithful to deliver them if they really want freedom. He promises to make a way of escape from any temptation, even smoking, if we call upon Him for aid (1 Cor. 10:13). As with any other request, we've got to be honest with ourselves and God.

The intestines are another organ of elimination. They eliminate the waste products from the food we eat. Once you have made use of most of the nutrition in the food you eat, the residue left goes through the small intestines where any more nutrition can be extricated. Then, in the large intestine, the residue forms a solid bulk. From here, if everything else is functioning normally, it passes out of your body.

Normally speaking, it is good for you to have a bowel movement every day, preferably in the morning after breakfast. Not everyone, though, lives a normal life today and so sometimes it's helpful to stimulate your intestinal tract naturally. A very excellent way to do this is to squeeze the juice of one lemon into a glass of warm water and drink it. Do this when you wake up in the morning, before breakfast, not during or after. Drinking this lemon juice in water first thing in the morning has a cleansing effect on your intestinal system. In addition to this, when your evening meal comes around, be sure to eat some raw vegetables with fiber in them. Vegetables such as lettuce, celery or cabbage and many others that have bulk in them are excellent. This is excellent for your bowels and acts as a broom to sweep out the substances that remain in the lower gastrointestinal tract.

Laxatives, in general, are not good to use. The reason is that they work on an irritation principle. They are designed to irritate the lining of your intestines and your intestines will react to this. Actually it is as if your intestines were to say, "Let's get rid of this because it's irritating us." Now, natural fiber or cellulose that comes from eating various raw vegetables and whole grains serves the same purpose without irritating the intestinal lining. It doesn't always work as fast, but works on a principle of stimulating the intestines rather than irritating them. This enables you to get the waste residue from your food out of your body in a natural way.

There are a lot of commercial products today that advertise high fiber content. That may be true, but be sure you read the label and examine the source of the fiber content. This may come as a surprise to you, but there's actually one bread company that uses ground up wood in its bread to help provide bulk in the intestinal tract! They call it fiber. When you read the label, however, it's called methacellulose, and that's nothing more than a fancy name for sawdust. Yes, it does provide you with bulk but certainly doesn't offer any nutritional value. This also allows them to advertise that they have fewer calories too, because wood does have fewer calories; it has no food value at all.

Pure water is an odorless, tasteless liquid made up of

hydrogen and oxygen that is more vital to most people's systems of cleansing and elimination than they realize. One of its most important functions is its use through your kidneys. Very much of the waste matter in your body is eliminated through your kidneys. Drinking plenty of good, filtered water is very important in the care of your kidneys.

When I talk about water, remember you shouldn't drink it with your meals, and you shouldn't drink ice cold water. Ice water tastes good on a hot day, but it actually shocks your vital internal organs upon contact, especially if you're overheated. For this reason, you'll never see a basketball or football coach give his players ice water. Even if you're served ice water in a restaurant or from a refrigerated drinking faucet, it's best to keep it in your mouth until it warms up a bit before letting it go down. For the best digestion to occur, you should drink liquids before a meal or not until a few hours after the meal.

Water stimulates the kidneys, and the kidneys eliminate waste materials from your body. When a patient comes to a physician, we usually take a sample of his urine. From the tests we run on the urine, we can determine whether it carries any infection and learn if other conditions may be present. However, this does not necessarily tell us the condition of the kidneys. A urine test can tell us what is coming away from the kidneys, but not what remains in the system. To find this out, we run another test on the blood to detect the amount of urea-nitrogen that remains and then we form a true index of how the kidneys are actually performing. This is how we make sure these vital organs are functioning up to par.

My friend who is a specialist in genitourinary diseases heads up a department in a large Los Angeles hospital. We traveled home together from a medical seminar held out West. Since he was a specialist in this field, I asked him what he did most often for kidney infections. Before he would answer me, he asked what procedures I followed. I explained some of my methods for stimulating kidney action, such as the use of antibiotics and so forth. When I had finished, he said to me, "This may surprise you, but I have seldom ever needed to resort to any drugs to stimulate the kidneys to get them working correctly. All I have to do, in most cases, is to get my patients to drink at least two quarts of water a day. If I can get them to do that, and keep on doing it, while they stop doing what had caused the infection to begin with, I usually clear them up without any medication at all!"

This has proven to be a very good plan. Most people don't drink enough water. According to my specialist friend, he has his patients drink two quarts, or the equivalent of a tall glass of water every two hours throughout the day. You'll find that if you drink this amount of water you can correct many so-called kidney conditions and keep your kidneys wholesome and healthy.

Many will say, "If I drink water, I keep it in my system. My ankles swell or I put on weight. I'll need a water pill." When people have swelling of the ankles it's invariably due to the fact that they are using some product to which they are allergic.

God has wonderfully contructed us with these cleansing systems in our bodies. Even so, we're living in an age when we have to be more careful in many ways about the things we put into our bodies. There are so many things in our environment today that weren't a real problem several generations back. Fumes from industrial centers and exhaust emissions from cars pollute the atmosphere, while pesticides and chemical fertilizers are used in such vast quantities that it's impossible to entirely escape from their effects. Several hundred artificial food additives in commercially produced foods keep them from spoiling and enhance their appearance. Most of these are harmful to your body over a period of time because they clog up your systems of elimination. When is the last time you've bought an apple with a worm in it? I'm sure it's been some time. The reason is that commercially produced apple crops are sprayed so much with insecticides that a worm wouldn't have a chance to live in an apple any more. But if a worm won't live in it, how good can it be for you? These insecticides are used on almost all fruits and vegetables. Simply washing them under the tap isn't going to get the residue off completely. These things are not terribly harmful in small amounts, but over a period of time they accumulate and are detrimental to our health.

One way to remove the spray residue on fruits and vegetables, if you can't buy them from an organic health food store, is to buy a biodegradable liquid cleaner. Make sure it is biodegradable. "Biodegradable" means the sudsing and cleaning agents in it will be broken down naturally into simple compounds when they are carried away by water. This does not pollute our streams and waterways with sudsing and chemicals. The Amway Company makes one called LOC, but there are other organic cleaners that are biodegradable. When you purchase your fruits and vegetables, take them home and place them in a bowl filled with a solution of LOC or other such biodegradable products and water. Let them sit there for a little while, then rinse them off with tap water. This will get most of the insecticide spray residue off the surface skin of the fruit or vegetable. Of course, a fruit with a thick skin that you peel before eating like a banana or an orange—does not require this, for the skin protects these fruits. That's one reason these types of fruits, vegetables and such—anything that you can peel off the skin to eat—are good to buy when you're traveling and can't adequately prepare your own food. The skin of these protects them to a degree. Nuts with the shells left on and hard boiled eggs are a few other good things to eat when on the road.

You can prevent the use of insecticides and sprays in your

own garden, if you have one, by using a solution of plain soap and water. I discovered this several years ago. Just make a rich soapy solution of soap and water. Again, though, use a biodegradable detergent. Spray this on all of your flowers, fruits and vegetables, and you'll discover that the bugs will keep away from them. I tried this on some flowers we had in our back yard. There were some bugs pestering them, and I sprayed the flowers with this soapy water solution, and they stayed away. They don't like the taste of it and we were able to completely get rid of these bugs by giving frequent sprays from this solution without harming the plants, the environment or ourselves.

We have to keep our bodies clean and we have to keep the organs God has endowed us with for the cleansing of the body as free from foreign impurities as possible. When we observe these natural laws of sanitation, we're helping to keep this "temple" in which we live clean. It might not make us more godly, but it certainly will keep us healthier.

10

LAWS OF ACTIVITY

You'll remember chapter 5's illustration of the shape of a
cross or four spokes of a wheel. Two of those spokes—two sides
of the cross—represent the areas of your life called work and
play. When these two aspects of your needs are kept in balance
with the other two major areas of your life—God and
love—your life will spin in an emotional balance, no matter
how fast you go. Many people get enough exercise through the
type of work they do; but other people today have to work in
more sedentary careers. Because they don't get exercise in their
work, they have to get it through some type of play or they have
to discipline themselves enough so that they incorporate it into
their daily schedule someplace.

You need to strengthen and keep strengthening the muscles of
your body all the days of your life. This is what I mean by the
natural laws of activity. To enjoy good health it is important for
you to get enough exercise to keep the muscle tone of your body
in a healthful condition. The purpose of exercise is to stimulate
the circulation of your blood throughout your body, increase
your breathing capacity, and strengthen the muscles in a
particular area. By this I do not mean that you start to lift
weights or begin to run five miles a day. Not at all. In fact too

much exercise can be as dangerous, if not more so, than too little exercise. It is important to remember that all exercise must be according to your needs and your ability.

I was at a medical seminar held in Miami, where I learned of two people dropping dead with heart attacks from jogging. A little over a year ago a well-known professional football player made the headlines when he dropped dead of a heart attack during pre-season workout practice. Jogging is fine; strenuous calisthenics are fine—if the person is conditioned for it and physically fit. These people who died stressed themselves too much. They worked out too hard, and the result was instant death.

Years ago, it was believed that when a person suffered from a heart attack and survived, he wasn't to do any form of strenuous activity. Exercise was out. But today cardiologists are administering "stress tests" to their patients who have had heart attacks to determine the extent of exercise that would be good for them to aid in their recovery. It would be good if everyone could take some form of a stress test to determine what type and how much exercise would be good for them, whether they've had a heart attack or not. We all have different endurance limits, oxygen intakes and metabolic rates. A stress test by a physician or physiologist can determine the amount of stress you can take. The doctor can then design an exercise program tailored especially for you. If possible, this is the best way to start off any exercise program.

When I was a young man, I regained my health by wrestling. I belonged to a wrestling club, and it was extremely beneficial to my developing strength and health as a young man. I worked out at this sport for years as a youngster, and even though I weighed only 135 pounds at the time, I was able to throw an opponent who weighed up to 200 pounds. During this period I also lifted weights and worked out with barbells and such. Yet today most of my exercise is in the form of walking.

The clinic I run is eighty feet long, forty feet wide and has thirteen different rooms. Daily I make dozens of trips up and down those halls, while I am working in my office. Also I live on a five-acre tract of land with a lake surrounded by trees. In the evenings or mornings I often walk around this area. Although I have an exerciser, and use it in a limited way, I don't do any strenuous calisthenics. I also have a whirlpool bath I use for exercise a couple of times per week. Basically all of my exercise is accomplished through walking. You must learn to exercise according to your age and ability and not according to someone else's preconceived idea of good exercise.

I've learned a great deal from my dog as far as exercise is concerned. My dog runs hard every so often. I let him out in the morning and he tears out, bursting with energy. After he runs around for a while, he comes in and drops down like a wet dish rag. He just lets go, flops down and relaxes. After all exercise there must be a form of relaxation to help you get benefit from what you do. The Bible speaks about this when it uses the term "temperance." Christians are to be temperate in all they do. "Temperance" means not doing anything that is wrong, and not overdoing anything that is right. This applies to exercise, eating and living in general.

A good way to temper your exercise program, no matter what it may be, is to finish in a relaxing posture. I discovered this while observing Olympic athletes work out. In their training program, you often see them lie on their backs at the completion of a workout session and prop their feet up against a tree or a wall. Elevating the feet above the head causes the flow of blood and circulation to increase in the head and brain area. The blood has been pumping itself to the parts of the body where the greatest strain has been applied. By propping the feet up, it now returns to the brain and this causes a refreshing feeling to occur. Even if you don't exercise like an Olympic athlete, this is a good relaxing posture for you to assume, daily.

Many mammals which have a history of longevity spend a good portion of their lives resting with their heads lower than their hearts. Now, it can't be verified scientifically that this is the reason for their longevity, but it's a valid observation. By propping your feet up for several minutes a day the circulation to your brain and head will increase. This is always a refreshing experience.

I believe it will also help prevent arteriosclerosis, hardening of the arteries in the brain at old age, the chief cause of senility. I have one patient who is over ninety years old who has been doing this for years. He claims it's helped his mental acuity very much and given him relief from a lower back problem too. I recommend it highly as a relaxing exercise to temper any program exercise. Just recline and put your feet up against a wall or a door for two to five minutes and you'll reap some very good benefits. I also recommend this for elderly people who might not have any form of exercise. It's a simple, safe way to increase brain and head circulation.

There are people who are intemperate in their sleeping. They spend more time in bed than they should. There are others who are intemperate in their working, and don't get enough rest. There are many people in our country today who are intemperate in their eating; they eat too much. There are also people who don't eat enough, who are trying to keep their bodies slim while undermining their health. Remember, the meaning of "temperance" is not doing anything that is wrong, and not overdoing what is right. You must practice temperance in all that you do.

I've known Christians who were intemperate in their church going. Yes, there are those who don't go enough, but there are some cases when people attend too much, as in the case of one lady who attended one of the churches I pastored. This dear sister spent so much time in church that she neglected her family and husband at home. She felt that her husband was very cruel to her because he didn't want her going to church all the time. She was determined to be there whenever the doors opened. It got to the point where her husband was threatening to leave her if she didn't stop going to church so much. Of course, she thought she was doing the righteous thing, but when I looked into the matter, I found out she was at fault. She had neglected to take care of her husband. She had neglected to prepare food for him and the children. She had neglected to wash and clean and manage the house. Her home was a shambles because of her neglect. Her church going became a cloak of rebellion, and she therefore became intemperate in it. With exercise, eating or any facet of life it is important to maintain a temperate attitude.

Before closing this section, I would like to issue a warning about a very prevalent type of exercise that has been lauded as having wonderful physical and emotional benefits. It is very definitely to be avoided—the system of Yoga. Yoga is offered on television, it's taught in Y.M.C.A.s and community centers across the land, and always the instructors say, "Yoga is not a religion. It's only a form of exercise and relaxation." This claim is absolutely and patently false. Yoga is a form of Hinduism. Make no mistake about it.

Even though Yoga has many physical benefits or what they term "asanas," it is still based upon a system of Hindu mystical and ascetic philosophy. It is impossible to practice Yoga without being caught up in its mystical overtones. Hatha yoga, which is the most popular type, starts in the physical realm and eventually leads the practitioner into the spiritual realm. Through certain physical and mental disciplines the person practicing Yoga is encouraged to withdraw from the world and meditate on spiritual principles or objects. It is not only physical exercise, no matter what any brochure may tell you. It is a Hindu discipline that tries to get a person to strive for a state of enlightenment in the spiritual realm.

This is how Christianity contrasts with every other religious system of the world. All of them, Yoga included, start with the physical realm and tell man that by doing certain things—withdrawing, physical discipline, special diet, meditation and rituals—he can attain to a spiritual reality and make contact with God. Christianity, however, is God coming to man and meeting him at his point of need.

This is the grace of God: "But God commendeth his love toward us, in that, while we were yet sinners, Christ died for us" (Rom. 5:8). We, as Christians, didn't have to discipline our minds and bodies to reach God. He reached down and drew us to himself just as we were. Then, after we were born again of His Spirit, we began to discipline and bring under subjection both our minds and our bodies. But He came to us first. We didn't work our way up to Him. This is Christianity. This is the love of God.

For this reason I caution people to stay away from Yoga, karate or any other form of physical exercise that is based upon a philosophical or religious foundation. Exercise, yes! But keep it simple and don't get involved in anything that promises you more than the stimulation of your circulation, the improvement of your breathing and the strengthening of muscles in your body. Find something designed for your needs and abilities. Above all, be temperate in all that you do.

11

LAWS OF NUTRITION

When I think of the influence America has had upon the nations of the world in terms of advanced technology, financial assistance, religious liberty, medical research, justice and plain old Yankee ingenuity, I hold my head high with pride and dignity. But when I, as a nutritionist, think of the influence our nation has had upon the eating habits of the world, I want to throw up my arms in dismay!

Don't misunderstand me. I'm very thankful to live in a land that has been able to help feed millions of people abroad who would have otherwise starved to death. But at the same time I've seen the results of changing the natural eating habits of a people from wholesome, native-grown crops to bottled soft drinks, candy bars and mass-produced refined foods with little or no nutritional value at all. Not only has our dietary influence proven to be detrimental to people abroad, but it has been causing a gastronomical feedback for generations here at home too.

The Eskimos are a people who, before American food began to permeate their culture, were able to live relatively healthy lives on a diet consisting mainly of whale blubber and fish. Scientists, who have studied this group of people, report that few problems resulted from their very limited diet. Certainly there were no cases of heart trouble or disease. Tooth decay was inconsequential in most of their lives. But then, as they developed a taste for American food, and started to eat it on a regular basis, they began to have all kinds of problems with their health—heart and teeth not excluded. Most of the American food they ate was processed food loaded with refined sugar and refined flour, not to mention a chemical feast of preservatives to which their bodies reacted adversely. Their disease rate increased. It is no longer a matter of conjecture; it is a proven fact that many of the diseases we have today are the direct result of the food we eat, and the way we eat it.

Metabolism is a process whereby the body takes nutritive materials and changes them into protoplasm—the physicochemical basis of all living matter. Metabolism is the process that converts what we eat and drink, breathe and think, into nutrition to feed and nourish our bodies. There are many things that come into our bodies through our senses and our minds that affect our health. Therefore, metabolism involves more than just the nutritive changes that take place when we eat food. It involves all that we eat and drink, breathe and think which feeds and nourishes our bodies.

When a patient comes to me because of metabolic or glandular problems, I always try to find out something about his genetic background. I try to find out what food his ancestors ate and how they prepared it. This is difficult when people are not able to trace their ancestry. For example a person may be the grandson of a Scotch-Irish man who was married to a woman from India with children born in all parts of the world. In cases like that it's difficult to obtain the necessary information. Nutritionally speaking, all of us are like the Eskimos. Before the twentieth century's technocratic society developed, most of our ancestors ate food that was naturally grown from the areas in which they lived. The formation of their genetic structures came partially from the nutrients in the food they ate. This has been passed down to you and me through generations. It's part of your genetic memory that we discussed in the first chapter. If an Eskimo came to me for assistance, the first thing I would encourage him to do is get back on a diet of fish and whale blubber if possible, while eliminating the wrong things he has been eating. Experience tells me his health would improve.

There's a popular proverb, "One man's meat is another man's poison." Metabolically speaking, this is certainly true. Because the people of a certain country or given area eat, enjoy and thrive on a certain food doesn't mean that same food would be good for you or me. One nutrition expert has observed that any change in dietary habits in less than 100 years becomes a crisis to the metabolism of the person making the change. When your diet becomes radically different from what you and your ancestors have eaten, your body rebels for a time to the change. Often this rebellion is manifested in the form of allergies and such and affects the health of the individual.

America is a melting pot of different cultures and races. As a result, we have adopted the dietary habits of many people. Yet by genetic background we are not at all the same. So if we all eat much the same food, we may find our metabolisms disordered and reactions may occur that we do not understand. Once I had a lady patient who was a full-blooded Cherokee Indian. She was a writer and an artist who had written many books on Indian language and culture. From time to time she would bring certain diets or food articles to me and want to know what I thought about them. I'd tell her, "Forget it. You need to eat the types of food your ancestors ate. You need to eat meat like jerky. You need to eat beans and corn. You'll never feel your best until you are eating food that is native to your ancestry because genetically, you are still tied with them."

My grandfather was born, lived almost a hundred years, and died in the same community. He visited other communities but he always returned to his home soil that was truly mother earth to him. The minerals, the soil, and the water were a part of his forefathers for about a hundred years and these became a part of him. When he became thirsty, his body yearned for the minerals found in the water from his well. His body desired food grown on the home farm. He never had any metabolic problems except when he would leave home and alter his eating habits by drinking different water, and eating different foods grown on soil that did not match his own chemical and mineral nature.

This is not true for most of us today. Few of us remain at our place of birth that we might absorb the chemicals and minerals from which our genetic lineage comes. Today we buy potatoes grown in Maine or Idaho. We eat eggs from the Carolinas, meat from the West, grain from the wheat fields of Iowa, vegetables from California and Florida, and berries from the East Coast. Nevertheless, I am convinced that if each of us followed our own genetic dietetic bent, and, as closely as possible, ate the same foods our ancestors did, we would be much better off.

Some time ago the crew of the Pueblo, a U.S. Navy ship, were captured by the North Koreans and fed the diet of their captors. However, this diet was not suitable for the American sailors. Many of them suffered intestinal upsets from the same diet their captors thrived on. The same may be said about American soldiers captured by the Japanese during World War II. When people have adjusted to a particular diet over a period of time, their bodies adapt to the specific food regimen. Strangers who come into a group or clan experience a difficult time, but after several generations they make the adjustment to a new dietary system.

Just because one food is good for a particular person does not necessarily mean it will be good for all. However, it will be good for people with the same genetic background. This helps to explain why the Italian colony living in Roseto, Pennsylvania, experiences less heart trouble than their American neighbors who follow the same diet.

Some observers have said it's because of their mental attitude. This may be partly true; however, I believe the greatest factor relates to the fact that the Italians adhere to their ancestral diets and ways. Their bodies have had sufficient time to adjust, even though we might not think of pizza and spaghetti as the basis for a good diet.

The Bantus of Africa have a simlar history. They have a very low incidence of arteriosclerosis, yet their diet would not indicate this. They have had centuries to adjust to their eating habits.

Once I was lecturing on this subject. One of the surgeons in the class came to me later and said, "Now I know why I like to eat fish three times a day." This surgeon's parents came from the Falkland Islands off the coast of northern Scandinavia, where their diet consisted mainly of fish. They also had some potatoes and a few vegetables. "My friends think there's something wrong with me because I like to eat fish so much, but now I know there isn't. I feel best when I'm eating plenty of fish."

You should try to learn exactly what your genetic background is, what your ancestors ate, and the way they prepared it. I realize this may be difficult in some cases, but you'll be helping yourself by learning as much as you can about the dietary customs of your people and trying to adhere to them as closely as possible. This will help you avoid some of the pitfalls that cause so many people in our nation to have gastric upsets.

There is a tremendous increase in metabolic disorders and diseases today. Through advertising, we are being shaped into a nation of people who eat about the same breakfasts, lunches and dinners. Perhaps in another hundred years or so we may all be able to get along on the typical American diet if it remains as it is now. But for your own health's sake now, you should try to adhere to the genetic-dietetic background of your ancestors.

Refined Manners But Not Refined Foods!

It's an asset to have refined manners, but a real detriment to your body to eat refined foods. This is another reason why most of your ancestors didn't have some of the metabolic imbalances we suffer today. They weren't exposed to processed, refined foods. I can still recall how my grandfather used to go to the mill with his sack of corn, wheat—or buckwheat when it was in season—and have it ground into flour. Then he'd take it home, and it would be baked into delicious and nutritious breads and cereals. But after a week or so the same process would have to be repeated because the weevils and other insects would get into the stone-ground flour despite every precaution. It just wouldn't last long on the shelf. Today all this has changed. We have flour that will last on the shelf for a long time without any spoilage because it's been so demineralized and degermed that it will not support life properly, even insect life. They won't eat it—but we do!

Around the turn of the century when I was born, there was not any refined flour or refined sugar on the market in our part of the country. I can remember going to the store, as a small child, and seeing the merchant scoop raw sugar from a large barrel and weigh it for me. Then around 1907, my mother discovered something new on the market shelves. She called it "processed" or "patented" flour. Today we call it "refined." The same thing happened to sugar during that period. Raw sugar gave way to refined sugar just as natural, stone-ground wheat gave way to refined flour. My mother liked these products because they were easier to work with and they lasted longer. On the surface they seemed like great innovations and improvements for the homemaker, but the underlying reality has brought a nutritional calamity to our country.

The millers started to make these refined products for two reasons. They discovered they could sell the by-products of the refining process. For example, when wheat was stone-ground there was no removal of the germ or the bran. It was sold as one product and had all the nutrients available to sustain life. The Bible refers to it as the staff of life—and it truly was. When they started to remove the germ and the bran, they discovered they could sell these items separately. The wheat germ could be sold to drug manufacturers. The bran could be sold to livestock producers. In other words, they could now sell several products: flour, wheat germ and bran instead of just stone-ground wheat. The second reason, as we already mentioned, is that it would last longer on the shelf. Economically, these reasons were very sound. Nutritionally, they were a disaster.

Today most of our packaged, commercial flour is what they call "enriched" or "fortified" flour. This is a misnomer. In fact, it's a downright joke. When they mill the wheat today they mill out all of the nutritive elements of the whole grain. By the time the refining process is completed the flour will virtually not support life!

Several years ago, before refined flour was "fortified," there was a research scientist who ran some experiments with refined flour and rats at a state university in the East. She had two groups of rats. One group she fed only water. The other group she fed water and refined flour. The group that had water only lived longer than the group that had refined flour and water! She notified the manufacturers and this and other studies led them to replace what they had taken out out of the flour with synthetic, chemical vitamins and nutrients to bring the flour up to a level that would support life in terms of the minimum daily requirements. Once they did this, they had the audacity to call the new product "enriched" or "fortified," making it sound as if the new product was better than the natural product itself! The millers take over twenty life-supporting elements from their so called "enriched" or "fortified" flour. Then they replace these with a few, chemically synthesized nutrients to bring it up to a minimal level for supporting life. The result is what you get when you buy refined flour or products such as most packaged breads made from refined flour.

When Jesus told us to pray, "Give us this day our daily bread" (Matt. 6:11), He certainly wasn't referring to the lifeless loaves of soft, white, "enriched" bread lining our supermarket shelves. Don't be deceived—any product that is made with "fortified" or "enriched" flour is not good for you. This includes most packaged breads, cereals and pastries.

The same is true of refined sugar. I remember hearing a missionary tell of the filthy methods of production of raw, natural sugar in underdeveloped nations. Although this may be true, you can remove the contaminants and still leave in the nutritive elements. What Americans use for sugar is that lovely-to-look-at, white, granulated cane sugar which is pure carbon. You know what carbon does to an automobile engine; it corrodes it and has to be systematically removed for better operation. That's precisely what refined sugar does to your blood vessels on the inside. The carbon process of sugar is just as destructive to your blood vessels as carbon is to a car.

Most Americans have a sweet tooth. This is because so many of the processed, refined foods they buy have sugar in them. Nearly a generation has been raised on these packaged goodies. It's been estimated that the average adult American eats between one hundred and one hundred and thirty pounds of sugar per year! Sounds incredible, doesn't it? It is true! Simply read the labels of the canned goods, cereals and store-bought packaged products, and you'll find nearly every one of them contains sugar. There are packaged cereals on the market today that are made with over 50 percent sugar. This sugar is the principle cause of tooth decay. It's also been connected to obesity, diabetes and heart disease.

The fact is that you really don't need to eat refined sugar at all. A well-balanced diet consists of natural sugars found in fruits, vegetables and grains. When you eat these foods, your body converts them into natural sugars or starches. This is more than adequate to supply your body's need for sugar without doing it any harm. When I take people off sugar, they usually have a very hard time for the first few days. They even feel sick sometimes because their bodies have become addicted to refined sugar, and they're experiencing a type of withdrawal.

Alcohol, for example, is made from sugar and grains fermenting together. When a person eats refined foods containing wheat and sugar, his body actually forms or generates its own alcohol. When this happens, problems develop. Even though you don't get drunk, it becomes difficult for you to break your addiction to it in the same way an alcoholic has a hard time breaking his habit. It's hard for you to ao without this artificial stimulant in your system.

If you feel you have to use a sweetener, use either raw honey or blackstrap molasses. Even an artificial sweetener is better than refined sugar. Refined sugar has no food value at all. Make sure the honey you buy is raw and hasn't been strained or pasteurized. Remember, though, that honey is a sweetener and even the Bible says, "It is not good to eat much honey" (Prov. 25:27).

The same is true with the molasses you buy. Read the label and make sure it hasn't been refined or "desulphurized." Blackstrap molasses is actually the waste product from refined sugar. It contains all the vitamins and iron that have been taken out to make that pleasant-looking white substance people like to sprinkle over their food. Actually, if you combined refined sugar with the blackstrap molasses, you'd end up with what was the original product before man tampered with it.

You should begin to cultivate less dependence on sweeteners. I know that's hard for many people, but it's absolutely essential to physical health. Many pediatricians today are beginning to tell mothers not to give sugar or products made from it to their children for the first couple of years of life so the children don't develop a dependence on this very sweet and deadly substance. And make no mistake about it, that's exactly what it is.

One of America's leading heart specialists, a doctor who has waited upon many world-famous people, including one of our presidents, is reported to have said recently that he never saw a patient with a heart infarct during his internship and early medical practice. This specialist is a senior citizen so he's referring to many years ago. He said he believed the reason for this was that people didn't eat as many refined foods then as they do today. He didn't just single out sugar as the culprit, but he associated it with the entire spectrum of refined foods today that satiate the American public.

Dr. John Yudkin, head of the Cardiac Division of Queens College Hospital in London, England, has written many articles on sugar and health in medical journals and a very thorough book entitled, *Sugar: Chemical, Biological & Nutritional Aspects of Sucrose*. In these works he really brings to light the harmful effects of sugar on the human body. I had the privilege of visiting with Dr. Yudkin while I was in England once, and I asked him how he started his research. He told me that he observed that the countries using the greatest amounts of sugar were the nations with the highest incidence of heart problems. He began to investigate this phenomenon by questioning people who were hospitalized with heart attacks about their diets—especially their use of sugar. He discovered a deadly parallel. The more sugar they used, the more heart trouble they had. I have observed this to be true. Refined foods, especially sugar, are detrimental to your health.

One time I was conducting a series of evangelistic meetings in the South and a woman, who was diabetic, came to me for prayer. She asked me to pray that she would be healed so she could eat anything she wanted. I told her I couldn't pray for her in that manner, but I would pray that the Lord would give her the wisdom to stop eating the things that were bad for her and start eating the foods that were beneficial to her. God won't do for us what we can do for ourselves.

When we learn of things that are detrimental to us, we must take authority over them and resist them. God doesn't want you to continue to sin against your body once you know principles of good nutrition. Remember, "sin" is "missing the mark," and when we discover sin in our lives, we should "Go and sin no more, lest a worse thing come unto thee."

I'm sure many of you are asking, "Dr. Miller, what in the world can I eat now that you've instructed me to remove all refined foods from my diet—especially refined sugar and wheat products?" I'm sure you feel like the fellow who was suffering from a severe obesity problem and came to me for aid. After I restricted his diet severely by giving him much of the information I'm passing on to you, he said, rather wryly, "Dr. Miller, do I take this diet before or after my meals?"

The truth of the matter is that once you begin to condition yourself with proper mental affirmations about correct eating and visualize yourself as establishing only natural and healthful eating habits, it's not so bad. This is where bringing your mind and body into subjection comes into play. You can visualize yourself avoiding any junk food, becoming the healthful, wholesome and fit person the Lord created you to be. But remember it's you—the real you, the hidden man of the heart—that has to do this. When you bring your mind and body into subjection to your spirit by observing these rules, better health is inevitable.

Shopping in a health food store is good if you can do it, but I realize some of you won't have access to one. Even if you don't have a health food store nearby, there are many good things you can buy in a supermarket. Remember this rule of thumb: if God made it, and man hasn't tampered with it, it's okay for you to eat. With the growing awareness of the nutritional deficiencies in our mass-produced foods, many supermarkets are opening up health food sections.

Let's look around a typical supermarket and see what you can buy. In the produce department any fruit or vegetable is good for you. You've learned how to clean these fruits and vegetables with a biodegradable liquid cleaner; now begin to enjoy them. Think of all the things you can find there. Nuts, figs, dates, raisins, plums, apples, bananas, oranges, grapefruits, melons and any other fruit in season. There are all sorts of vegetables: green peppers, lettuce, celery, radishes, spinach, squash, peas, potatoes, beans, zucchini, turnips, carrots, cabbage, mushrooms, tomatoes and many other vegetables. (Incidentally, if you are fond of salads, there are recipes for natural salad dressings without chemicals.) Learn to eat raw vegetables and fruits. The less cooking, the better for you.

Then there are poultry, meats, fish, cheeses and eggs. Some stores are carrying a line of natural, whole-grain breads without preservatives. Just be sure to read the labels. You will want to avoid refined flour and refined sugar as much as possible, as well as products made with these.

You might have to go to a health food store to get your raw

honey and to replace the refined flour. There you can get some whole wheat flour, rice flour or soy bean flour and other natural whole grains.

You don't have to starve yourself to death. Simply begin to buy food that is close to its natural state and hasn't been processed by man. You can do it and you can begin to enjoy it. One other great help in shopping is to break yourself of impulsive buying. Don't buy products because they are advertised as "easy to prepare" and convenient. This is where the whole vicious cycle of refined and processed foods began. Take time with your food—both in buying and preparing it. Believe me, it won't be wasted time.

One of the reasons for eating fruits and vegetables primarily raw is that they supply more vitamins and minerals in the raw state. When they are cooked, canned or frozen, many vitamins and minerals are destroyed. DNA (deoxyribonucleic acid) and RNA (ribonucleic acid) are found in every living thing. They are found in your body. They are also found in fresh fruits and vegetables, but when these foods are cooked, DNA and RNA are destroyed along with vitamins and minerals.

When you eat these foods raw, you will reap the full benefit of these two very important elements as they stimulate their counterparts in your body. Fresh fruits and vegetables, as mentioned earlier, also have a purifying effect on your intestines and help remove toxic things in your system. Learn to experiment with vegetables and fruits. Many vegetables you've been used to eating only when they were cooked, will have a good taste when they are served raw in a salad. Spinach, mushrooms or certain soft-skinned squash like zucchini can be cut up into a salad. When you cook vegetables, cook them only briefly. Also cook them in waterless cookware, if you can, or steam them, and you'll retain much of their nutritional value.

It may interest you to know what foods are mentioned in the

Bible as fit for human consumption. Here is a list taken from *The Texas Herald*:

Apples (Joel 1:12)	Figs (Num. 13:23; Mark 11:12-13)
Grapes (Deut. 23:24)	Pomegranates (Num. 13:23)
All Fruits (Gen. 1:29)	Palm Dates (Lev. 23:40)
Herbs (Gen. 1:29)	Olive Oil (Lev. 2:4; Lev. 8:10)
Olives (Deut. 8:8)	Corn (Ruth 2:14; 1 Sam. 17:17)
Wheat (Ps. 81:16)	Roasting Ears (2 Kings 4:42; Lev. 2:14)
Bread (Luke 22:19)	Salt (Lev. 2:13; Mark 9:50)
Barley (Ruth 2:23)	Pottage (Stew) (2 Kings 4:38)
Honey (Ps. 81:16)	Milk (Isa. 7:21-22)
Butter (Isa. 7:22)	Cheese (1 Sam. 17:18)
Goat's Milk (Prov. 27:27)	Locust, Grasshoppers (Lev. 11:22; Mark 1:6)
Almonds (Gen. 43:11)	Nuts (Gen. 43:11)
Beef (Deut. 14:4)	Mutton (Deut. 14:4)
Goat Meat (Deut. 14:4)	Fish (John 21:9-13)
Eggs (Luke 11:12-13)	Venison (Deut. 14:5)

Certain meats from animals called unclean by God were from scavengers. As the Israelites wandered for forty years in the wilderness these scavengers ate the filth left by the Israelites, thus making them unfit for human consumption. It is my opinion that things are different now because such animals are raised in pens and under sanitary conditions. Therefore, these animals might safely be slaughtered and eaten by man.

Allergies

I did not discover I was allergic to both sugar and wheat

products—even whole wheat bread—until a series of tests were performed on me in the Salvatore Mundi Hospital in Rome, Italy. I used to retain water all the time and put on quite a bit of weight. In fact I was dangerously overweight, and it was beginning to affect my health. When I eliminated wheat products and sugar from my diet, I began to lose weight. I lost a total of seventy-five pounds in six months and I have never put it back on. This was many years ago.

Why was my diet so effective? My allergy had partially closed my kidneys so that if I ate an once of bread, I would gain a pound of weight! This seemed ridiculous to me when I first discovered it. Nonetheless, it was true, for it caused me to retain a pound or more of water when I drank. The water would stay in my system and make my ankles swell. This allergy to wheat products would cause the tubules of my kidneys to swell, making me unable to pass off the water I had taken in. In my practice I've discovered that people with swollen lower legs and ankles usually have this condition because they are eating something to which they are allergic. This almost invariably involves flour or wheat products. In other cases it involves sugar. Even if a person isn't allergic to sugar, he should eliminate it from his diet. I am allergic to both; therefore, I remove them from my diet. Many other people are also allergic to them, but they don't know it. Often I have told my patients to eliminate the use of these two substances, and this alone frequently takes care of their problem.

I would like to give you a simple method for determining if you are allergic to something. Allergies have become a serious problem in our country. They occur when you are sensitive to something that comes in contact with your skin, lungs or stomach. The reaction can take the form of itching, running of the nose, patches of skin breaking out, hives, canker sores, low blood pressure, epileptic seizures, dizziness, tiredness, constipation, gastric ulcers, headaches, depression, angioneurotic edema or any one of a dozen or more other symptoms. These symptoms can be caused by something you touch, breathe or eat.

One reason why allergies are becoming increasingly prevalent is that we are coming in contact with more irritants in the form of air pollutants, food additives, and insecticides than ever before. Many children today are becoming allergic to cow's milk. This may be due to substances sprayed on the cow or what the cow's food is treated with, or injections the animal receives. Some people have been found to be allergic to the aluminum in utensils used for preparing or storing it. Many underarm deodorants contain aluminum, and I have treated many women with underarm irritation from this. There are also some baking powders that contain aluminum and these cause gastric upsets and intestinal irritations including diarrhea. There are many substances today that may be affecting you; and simply by eliminating contact with them, you can improve your condition drastically.

Here's an easily applied test that you can perform at home to determine if you are allergic to anything. All that is required is a watch with a sweep second hand, and you're in business. When you awaken in the morning, take your pulse before rising. There are some kinds of materials we sleep on such as kapok or feathers or a synthetic fiber that may cause some trouble, but all things being equal, your pulse should be the lowest in the morning before you get out of bed. This establishes your norm.

Once you get up and resume your normal activities, your pulse will naturally rise. Check your pulse again right before breakfast. Then check your pulse one more time thirty minutes after breakfast. If your pulse rises ten beats per minute above the check you took directly before eating your meal, there is likely to be an allergy present. If your pulse rate doesn't increase ten beats per minute, you're probably safe in eating what you had for breakfast. But if it did rise ten beats or more, then you should start testing each item you had for breakfast separately to find the culprit. Once you discover it, eliminate it from your diet completely—you'll see symptoms disappear. This is a very easy way to determine an allergy, but remember it applies only to adults. Children usually have much faster pulses and the same scale shouldn't be used for them.

Do the same kind of testing with odors, things you touch or fumes you inhale. If your pulse rate doesn't go above eighty-four beats per minute at any time, then it is unlikely that you have come in contact with anything to which you are allergic. Take into account factors such as colds, fevers and infections which will cause your pulse rate to become more rapid. The pulse test is the most accurate and reliable method for the layman. It requires only a watch with a sweep second hand and some time.

I haven't delivered babies for a number of years, because with a very busy practice I can't find the time to leave an office full of patients to go deliver a baby. However, I still supervise the diets of pregnant women when they desire it, and I let someone else do the delivering. I make especially sure that the expectant mother gets a full complement of all dietary necessities plus a very needed supply of "trace minerals." These are minerals such as molydenum, chromium, selenium and others. Many doctors know very little about the effects of deficiencies of trace minerals in the pregnant woman, but I have found that when deficiencies exist, they will often show up in the child in the form of an allergy. When I have examined and treated people with allergies and investigated their cases thoroughly, I have frequently discovered they were born of a mother who was deficient in trace minerals during the time of pregnancy. The absence of these trace minerals in the mother often causes certain organs within the child to be incompletely developed. As the child grows, this manifests itself in the form of allergies.

Sea water offers the best source of all the trace minerals you'll ever need. It contains virtually every mineral of the earth in a dissolved form. If you live near the ocean and can arrange for someone to bring you back a bucket of sea water from about twenty-five miles out, and several fathoms deep, you would obtain a good source of trace minerals. Don't collect any sea water from along the coastlines, as this is often polluted with fertilizers and other chemicals from rivers dumping into the ocean. When you get the sea water, boil it for about ten minutes to get rid of the impurities. Then take a couple of tablespoons of it every day and you'll be supplied with all of the trace minerals you'll need. Of course, if you don't have access to the sea, you can find a natural trace mineral supplement at your health food store.

The Vitamin Question

It seems everybody talks about vitamins today, and there is much controversy in this area. But despite the controversy, vitamins are essential to good health. We need to take them because so much of our food has been processed to death and drained of its full vitamin and mineral strength. Also, as we have discovered, cooking vegetables and fruits lessens their nutritive content. It's also possible that the foods we eat may not have been raised on proper soil or with proper care. The length of time it takes to get from the fields to the market to your table also depletes the vitamin content of fresh fruits and vegetables. We just can't keep track of all these factors; therefore, it is important to have vitamin supplements in your diet. However, if we take them on a regular basis, the body won't require great amounts of them.

I don't intend to list every vitamin, explain its function and sources, or what symptoms may be present if it is lacking in one's diet. I've seen books that attempt to do that, thereby causing many people to try to diagnose their own symptoms and vitamin deficiencies. Since these people are not trained physicians, they often misjudge their symptoms, and the results can be harmful. When trying to determine what vitamins you need the most, the best method is to offer your body a virtual vitamin smorgasboard and let it make its own selection. A vitamin is really anything necessary for the growth and proper functioning of your body. Most vitamins your system doesn't need will be passed off through your organs of elimination. There are exceptions, but it is very rare for anyone to take an overdose of vitamins. Vitamin D is an exception, however, and there are some people who might be allergic to "massive" doses of it, so I wouldn't recommend too large a dose of it. The same is true of Vitamin A.

Years ago I developed a substance called LIVEC. It's sold in many health food stores. I assisted a vitamin manufacturer, The Enzyme Process Company of Northridge, California, with its development. It contains all the substances we know anything about: the DNA factors, the RNA factors, all of the vitamins and minerals, plus the amino acids and enzymes your body needs. By taking such a product, you allow your body to select what it needs and dismiss the items which are in surplus. This is the type of product I suggest you offer your system as a "vitamin smorgasbord."

I take plenty of vitamins. I have for years, and I partially attribute my good health to them along with the other factors I've mentioned. Don't be intimidated by the government measure referred to as MDR (Minimum Daily Requirement) or what is sometimes called the U.S. Recommended Daily Allowance, U.S. RDA. When dealing with nutrition you shouldn't be concerned with minimums—but maximums.

Some time ago we were beset with a siege of viral infections including influenza and pneumonia. I was treating people with these diseases all day long, day in and day out for weeks. What I did was take plenty of Vitamin C. I took capsules of 500 units of Vitamin C all day long. I kept one nearly constantly in my mouth while I went about the work of the day, and I didn't contract any viral diseases. No, I don't believe you can take too many vitamins, except in the cases of vitamins A and D.

Again, the best procedure is to take a full supplement and let your own system do the selection. Also, take them in their natural form—not synthetic vitamins. Some authorities say it makes no difference, but it does. Natural vitamins are the best. You can take a kernel of corn or a grain of wheat, for example. You can break down its chemical make-up in the laboratory and reproduce those exactly proportioned chemicals synthetically. But if you plant it, you can never make it grow! A synthetic substitute will never replace the natural one where vitamins are concerned. There is always something missing when man tries to improve on nature. He makes many noble attempts to do this, but it only takes a few years to realize the futility of such endeavors.

Some sixty years ago an uncle of mine moved from Ohio to Illinois. He once told me that when he first came to Illinois they grew corn, and fed it to their hogs to fatten them for market. As technology increased they learned ways to increase the yield of their corn by artificial, or synthesized, fertilization and a process known as hybridizing. Although this enabled them to get twice the yield from their corn in later years than they were able to sixty years previously, they discovered it took twice as much of this new corn to feed their hogs and get them fattened for market. They also had to add other livestock supplements. The yield had been increased, but the nutritional value had been cut in half! In recent years other experiments have verified my uncle's discovery about artificially increasing the yield from the soil. The nutritional content is cut in proportion to the artificially induced increase in yield. Even so, the practice is continued because things are sold on the market on the basis of volume and weight—not upon intrinsic nutritional value.

The same type of experiment was tried on chickens. I learned of this while I was attending a seminar on nutrition sponsored by a natural vitamin manufacturer in Iowa. The test involved two chickens hatched from the same group of eggs, with the same parents. One of the chickens was raised on natural grains without any artificial supplements. The other chicken was given hormones, antibiotics and other artificial supplements that have been used in feeding and aiding livestock for years. The one that received the artificial supplements did grow to be a bigger and fatter chicken. It also remained healthy throughout its life. When they butchered both chickens and macerated them by putting them through a process whereby all of the nutrient factors—the vitamins, minerals and so forth—were analyzed, they found that the bigger chicken was nearly twice the size and weight of the chicken that was allowed to grow and feed naturally. The amount of nutrition in the meat of both of these chickens was exactly the same! Again, chickens are usually sold by weight—not by nutritional value.

It seems to be one of God's natural laws that when man improves the volume, weight or amount of a crop or livestock by artificial means, the food value of that product is decreased in the same proportion. This is why I maintain we need to use vitamins—those that are naturally manufactured.

Ideally, you should be able to obtain all the vitamins you need through the sound eating habits you're learning about in this book. But even when you are following these guidelines, you can't always tell the nutritional content of the food you eat. For this reason, and others previously mentioned, I advise people to take a full vitamin supplement that will afford them three or four times the MDR or the U.S. RDA and allow their own bodies to make the selection for them.

What I'm sharing with you is the same information I have shared with other doctors at medical conferences and seminars throughout the world. I always desire to keep abreast of the latest developments in health so I can be of greater service to those I serve.

The Proper Order Of Eating

Now that we've discussed what you should and shouldn't eat, I'd like to talk to you about "how" you should eat, or the order of eating. This is neglected in most health books because the authors haven't really studied the physiology of digestion. But once you become aware of how your digestive system works, you'll see how much sense there is in learning to eat food in its proper order.

When you are born into this world, the first food you are exposed to is mother's milk. Milk is a protein source, and it's metabolized by the use of hydrochloric acid in your stomach. So, the first secretion that comes into your stomach at birth is hydrochloric acid. Hydrochloric acid metabolizes or digests protein. Throughout your life, whenever you eat anything, the first substance of secretion that comes into your stomach is hydrochloric acid. That's the way you're made. It's interesting to note that, originally, the word "protein" meant "that which comes first." I want you to remember that. Protein should be that which comes first in your order of eating. Why? Because hydrochloric acid is the first secretion that forms in your stomach, and it's designed to digest and metabolize protein first and best.

In addition to the hydrochloric acid that the baby's tummy

secretes, an enzyme called rennin comes forth also. This helps digest the milk too. However, the stomach stops producing rennin at about the age of six years. By that age the child eats many other foods to obtain nourishment so the rennin enzyme to digest milk isn't needed any more. This is one reason milk isn't really necessary for adults, because they don't produce the enzyme rennin to metabolize it properly. When your body ceases to produce rennin, it starts to produce pepsin. Now although milk isn't required in an adult's diet, milk products, such as cheese, yogurt and sour cream, are good. The chemical change from milk to cheese involves a process similar to what the rennin does in a baby's stomach, making cheese and other milk products easily digestible. But plain milk isn't the best for an adult.

Any and all other protein foods should be eaten first to meet that initial hydrochloric acid produced in your stomach throughout your life. Protein foods come from sources such as: meat, fish, poultry, cheese, yogurt, eggs, all seafood, most nuts and beans. These begin to be digested by hydrochloric acid in the stomach. Hydrochloric acid does nothing for starches, carbohydrates or even vegetables. So, if you eat a starch food first or a sweet food first, you may get a stomach ache or some form of indigestion.

When your body stops forming rennin, it forms pepsin. This enters your stomach after the hydrochloric acid, a process that continues throughout life. The hydrochloric acid is always followed by pepsin. Pepsin helps to digest most other foods like vegetables and fruits, *except* sweets and starches. Therefore, you should eat your protein first, your vegetables second and save your carbohydrates until last.

Carbohydrates include anything starchy such as cereals, wheat, rye, barley, most root vegetables and some fruits like bananas. Carbohydrates require an enzyme called ptyalin to complete their full digestion. This enzyme is found in saliva. It predigests carbohydrates before they enter the stomach. The final digestion of carbohydrates take place in the small intestine where other enzymes go to work. Ptyalin in the saliva is necessary to completely digest carbohydrates. This means you should always chew them thoroughly and slowly. This sets up the essential predigestive work. If carbohydrates are not chewed and mixed well with the saliva, they may cause gas to form in the stomach and cause indigestion. So always chew your carbohydrates thoroughly. In short, you should chew things like mashed potatoes and bananas much longer and more thoroughly than you chew meat. Hydrochloric acid will dissolve the meat, but the carbohydrates need the ptyalin of your saliva as a predigestive measure before they can be fully assimilated into your digestive system.

Each of these three major categories of food—protein, vegetables and carbohydrates—are digested by different secretions in the digestive process. This means that even though you may be eating a well-balanced diet, the order in which you eat is very important. If you will begin to eat in this order: proteins first, vegetables second, and carbohydrates last, you will be able to overcome many types of intestinal disorders. I have seen it work in thousands of cases, and I always prescribe this method to my patients. I have seen people relieved of indigestion, diverticulitis and even gastric ulcers simply by learning to eat in the proper order based upon the physiology of digestion. It will help with a host of dietary problems. I have had people tell me they couldn't eat anything with roughage in it, but when they began to apply this proper order of eating, they have found that they could.

You should try it for several weeks before you look for a definite change. Your system needs time to correct the improper order in which you have been eating for years. But you will notice a change, and you'll feel better as a result.

Even if you are eating a vegetarian meal, always start out with some protein first such as an egg, yogurt or even some nuts to meet that initial hydrochloric acid secretion that is designed for protein. When you go out to a restaurant, don't eat your salad first. Save it until after you eat some protein. Some sour fruits such as oranges, grapefruit, cherries, berries, tomatoes and apples are acidic in nature and can be eaten first in place of a protein, or with a protein.

Some people, especially the elderly, have some difficulty digesting protein. It may be due to wrong eating habits of the past. A good thing to do in such cases is to take a tablespoon of apple cider vinegar in a glass of water before sitting down to a meal. This will help reactivate the weakened hydrochloric cells. It also helps increase the potassium level of the tissues and actually helps to digest the protein itself.

"What about snacks?" you may be asking. In the first place, a starchy or sweet snack is not the right thing to take. If you're going to snack, take some protein or a piece of citrus fruit. Whole nuts that haven't been roasted or a piece of cheese would be better than a starchy or sweet snack. Protein means "that which comes first," so whenever you put anything into your stomach first, beginning a meal or a snack, make sure it's a protein food.

I know it's difficult to maintain this exact order of eating when certain dishes are served—such as a stew or a sandwich with several ingredients in it. Even in cases like this, always try to start by eating a protein appetizer because this will utilize the initial hydrochloric acid.

Some of you may have a drinking problem. I'm not referring to alcoholic beverages, however. I mean that many of you are drinking liquids with your meals. This is very bad to do. Recent research has revealed that harm can be done to your digestive system when you drink any liquid, with the exception of milk in moderation, during your meals. Water, tea, coffee, or fruit juices are not beneficial when they are drunk with your meals. Most of you know that oil and water don't mix. All you need to prove this is to place some water in a glass and pour some oil on top of it. The oil won't mix. It will float on top of the water. However, when you place oil in milk, it will mix. Therefore, milk can be tolerated in small amounts. But it's best not to drink any liquid with your meals. Here's why.

Most foods of a protein nature contain oils. These oils are needed for the body to help lubricate every part of it. Oil is important in the prevention of joints drying out, which happens to a lot of elderly people. Oil also helps prevent constipation, and it helps keep the body appearing youthful. There are many internal functions of the body that are affected by the lack of oil. Good sources of oil are most animal foods. Butter is one of the richest; so are fish oils, especially cod liver oil. Vegetable oils are useful, but not as good as the oils you get in eggs, butter and fish.

I know some of you will object when I tell you to eat things like eggs and butter. ''What about cholesterol?'' you may ask. The fact is that you need not be afraid of cholesterol occurring in any food that is natural. The cholesterol that builds up in the blood and is dangerous to your health is caused by refined carbohydrates, sugar and flour—starches that have not been fully metabolized in the liver. This happens because people don't eat in the proper order. The blood cholesterol build-up that is dangerous is caused by refined carbohydrates that are not fully metabolized. On the other hand, natural foods such as eggs are high in animal cholesterol, but they are also high in lecithin. The lecithin is very valuable to your body, and has a neutralizing effect on the cholesterol in the eggs. But the thing to understand is that cholesterol found in eggs and such is not the same cholesterol that is found in human blood.

I have eaten as many as five eggs a day for many years and have a cholesterol reading below 200 mg. per cent. That's considered low by all standards. I also eat butter and other naturally-occurring oily foods and have no trouble with my cholesterol count. Remember, our ancestors used natural lard and butter without any harm being done to them. So can we. Eskimos have lived on fish and whale blubber for years without any trace of heart trouble. Any natural food that is high in oil or animal cholesterol content will not hurt you. It is eating refined carbohydrates, eating in the improper sequence or order, and drinking liquids with your meals that is dangerous and causes problems. These are the things that cause improper metabolization in the liver and, as a result, form cholesterol in the human blood.

Water and oil certainly don't mix, especially in your body. When you drink water, coffee, tea or fruit juices with your meals, the oils in the food you have eaten are mixed with the water in these drinks and the result is that the oils are literally floated out of the digestive tract before they can be utilized. Fats and oils are supposed to be metabolized in the liver, but when they are floated out of the system before this can happen, they don't do you any good. Liquid, except for milk, moves through your system very rapidly. However, it takes up to three hours to digest a meal properly. So you should wait at least two or three hours if possible after your meals before you drink any liquid. This allows the digestion to be completed and the oils to be utilized and metabolized in the liver where bile is formed for this process. Do all your drinking before you eat—up to ten minutes before a meal—because liquid will pass through your system very quickly. Drink a glass of water first thing in the morning and squeeze into it the juice of one lemon. Drink plenty of water throughout the day.

Whenever possible, drink filtered water or natural spring

water. The latter is more expensive, but if you can't afford that, at least invest in an inexpensive water filter that you can attach to your faucet or spigot at home. You'll filter out many of the impurities that are found in tap water. Don't drink distilled water that has had all of the mineral content removed. Filtering your water takes the impurities out, but leaves the minerals in. And be sure to change your filter as often as needed.

If You Don't Watch Your Weight, Others Will.

I believe everybody has a beautiful body. Sometimes it's covered with fat so nobody can see it, but nonetheless, I believe everyone has a beautiful body. I know what it's like to be fat. As I shared earlier, for a good portion of my life I was overweight. When I discovered I was allergic to wheat products and sugar, and removed those items from my diet, I lost seventy-five pounds over a period of six months and have never regained it. I'm very thankful to God for this because it was affecting my health; and if you're overweight, it will affect you too. It will affect you both physically and emotionally.

There's a Scripture verse I like to use to help people who come to me for weight problems. I realize I'm using it out of context, but it becomes a kind of positive motto to help people maintain their proper weight. It's one more of those affirmations that helps the overweight person take dominion over his body. It reads, "But thou shalt have a perfect and just weight, a perfect and just measure shalt thou have: that thy days may be lengthened in the land which the Lord thy God giveth thee" (Deut. 25:15). This verse is really speaking about not cheating anyone, but I tell my patients to apply it to their own weights and measurements. Many report that it's been very helpful. So remember, if you want to lose weight, God wants you to have a perfect and just weight and measurement that you might enjoy better health.

Because of my studies in metabolism and endocrinology, I've had very good success in helping people get rid of fat. I've probably attended to over 6,000 people in the last twenty years who have had weight problems. In fact, my program for patients isn't called "weight control"; I call it "fat control." Literally, what I do with my patients, in addition to changing their diets and eating habits, is to give them glandular injections to help convert fat calories in their bodies into protein calories. The fat becomes protein. I use something imported from Sweden known as a "fat mobilizer."

You see, every pound of excess fat in your body contains 3600 calories. If you don't utilize all the calories you're eating, it will accumulate as fat in different parts of your body. On the other hand, every pound of protein in your body—everything other than fat—has only 1200 calories. By using this "fat mobilizer" through injections, a pound of fat is converted into a pound of protein and 2400 calories are used up each time. That's the difference between the 3600 calories in a pound of fat compared with 1200 calories in a pound of protein.

Even if a person doesn't lose weight, he loses inches. This method enables the patient to start using body fat as part of their diet. This is the same treatment that has been used successfully by movie stars and other celebrities who have weight problems. I have helped thousands of patients this way. But it's not magic! It will not work unless the person revolutionizes his eating habits in addition to the glandular injections.

People are fat because of three basic reasons: (1) they are eating more food than they need; (2) they're eating the wrong types of food; or (3) they're eating their food in the improper order. If you're healthy and you put on weight, it should be distributed evenly over your body. However, if you accumulate fat in different parts of your body, it has to do with a malfunctioning of your glands. If you put on fat around your hips, it's because your pituitary gland is not working as well as it should. If the fat piles up in your belly, that's because your thyroid gland isn't functioning properly. If your adrenals are not working well, you'll put on weight around the shoulder girdle of your body, the upper part of your torso. There are a number of glands controlling the excess weight. If you notice that you put on weight in specific areas, instead of evenly, it's a good indication your glands are not functioning the way they should. In such cases I would suggest that you consult with a metabolism expert or an endocrinologist who can probably help you in this area by restoring the proper working of your glands. Then the food will go to the places where it is intended and supply the needs of your body.

Let's assume you have a "normal" weight problem. By paying heed to the methods of diet and eating I've already discussed, you can greatly improve your condition. But you must be honest in answering these three basic questions: Are you eating more than you need? Are you eating the wrong types of food? Are you eating them in the improper order? Only you can answer these questions honestly.

If you want to lose weight, I'm going to give you a basic dietary regimen to follow that is guaranteed to help you lose weight and provide you with your daily food needs.

1. Don't eat anything with sugar or flour in it.
2. Don't eat fried foods. Cook, broil, boil or stew them.
3. Don't prepare your food using any oil, grease, lard, fat or butter. We want to use your fat instead of these.
4. Eat in the proper order: proteins first, vegetables second, and carbohydrates last. (However, the carbohydrates in this diet are eliminated.)

5. For breakfast eat a hard-boiled egg, one half grapefruit and a small portion of cottage cheese.

6. For lunch eat a medium-size portion of meat and a few vegetables.

7. For supper eat a small protein appetizer such as plain yogurt, a hard-boiled egg, etc. followed by a good selection of raw vegetables.

8. Drink plenty of water, up to two quarts a day, but not until at least a couple of hours after each meal.

If you keep on this diet, you will lose weight. There's no doubt about it. It's rigorous, but if you want to lose weight, you'll do it.

Man was created to eat a hearty breakfast because during the night the body tends to repair itself, thus depleting the blood sugar levels. A good-sized breakfast replenishes this. The work that follows breakfast expends the energy build-up from breakfast. When lunch arrives, a smaller portion is needed. Normally, this will be turned into energy during the afternoon. Your evening meal should be the lightest. This is the meal that many Americans make the largest and the things eaten during this meal usually turn into fat. Most people who are overweight have a habit of eating no breakfast, or a skimpy one, a light lunch and a heavy dinner. This is the worst pattern to follow, as research conducted by doctors and nutritionists at a large midwestern medical school has proven.

They took a group of volunteers and fed them all the same amount of food daily for a period of time. For the first period of days they fed them a good breakfast, a fair lunch, and then a light dinner. All of the people lost weight. Then they administered to them the same caloric proportion of food again over another period of days—only this time they skipped the breakfast and gave them a fair lunch with a heavy dinner incorporating all of the food they had previously eaten at breakfast. This time they all gained weight. In each period of days they had the same amount of food. By skipping breakfast and eating a heavy dinner, they all gained weight.

If you don't want to practice the rigorous diet I've prescribed, but you would like to cut down your weight slightly, start applying this principle. Eliminate your heavy evening meal. Instead, eat a good breakfast, a light lunch and light supper, preferably with plenty of raw vegetables. Someone has said that to lose weight you should eat like a king in the morning, a queen at noon, and a pauper at night. It works. Conversely, if you want to gain weight, simply reverse this order.

Fasting

As a believer in God's Word, fasting should become a normal part of your Christian experience. Jesus didn't say "if" you fast, but He said, "When ye fast" (Matt. 6:16). It is an expected discipline to be followed. The rewards are greatly given by our heavenly Father when a fast is conducted in the proper way with the right spiritual motives (Matt. 6:16-18).

The Bible presents many reasons to fast, ranging from spiritual strength to casting out demons. "Howbeit this kind goeth not out but by prayer and fasting" (Matt. 17:21). The people's fast changed God's mind concerning judgment: "The people of Nineveh believed God; and proclaimed a fast. . . . And God saw their works, that they turned from their evil way; and repented of the evil, that he had said he would do unto them" (Jonah 3:5, 10). We know the Lord Jesus began His earthly ministry after His baptism by John and was led of the Spirit into the wilderness where He fasted forty days, after which He was tempted of the devil, as recorded in the fourth chapter of Matthew. By and large, I believe the primary reason for a New Testament believer to fast is to bring his appetites and habits into subjection. Those appetites not only pertain to eating and drinking, but to any craving of the flesh, even sexual activity. "Do not cheat each other of normal sexual intercourse, unless of course you both decide to abstain temporarily to make special opportunity for fasting and prayer" (1 Cor. 7:5 Phillips). Fasting involves self-control, and its benefits are manifested in these three areas of our lives—spiritual, emotional and physical. There's no sense in taking authority over the devil in any area of your life if you can't take authority over your own fleshly desires of mind and body.

Having said that, I also want to say that for a believer to try to imitate what Jesus or Moses did in the way of a prolonged fast is extremely dangerous, and I do not recommend it at all. Just the other day I received some literature from a well-known Christian minister. He's had a problem with being overweight for some years and he's finally won the victory over it through fasting. His is a tremendous testimony, and I know he's encouraged many Christians to fast. This is all well and good. Christians should fast. However, he makes this very inaccurate deduction whereby he says that the average person can fast for as long as thirty or forty days without suffering any ill effects! This is patently untrue. There are many people who could not fast that long and should not even attempt to do so. People with a history of diabetes, thrombosis, or hypoglycemia should not fast. Elderly people should not fast, unless under the supervision of their physician, because the body doesn't replenish itself as rapidly in old age as it does when we're younger. This dear brother means well, but he's basing it upon trying to imitate what Christ did, rather than how the Holy Spirit would lead.

In Mark 1:12, it's recorded that the Spirit of God literally drove Jesus into the wilderness to fast forty days. It wasn't because it seemed like a good idea to Him. It wasn't because He wanted to purge his body from impurities or lose weight, which are some of the benefits of fasting. No, Jesus was driven by the Spirit to take on this prolonged fast. It didn't come about by reading literature on fasting. He was compelled by the Spirit of God to undertake this fast. And it's for this reason that I say as a doctor and a man who loves God with all my heart, that for any person to attempt a prolonged fast beyond seven to ten days without this extreme unction by the Spirit of the Lord as recorded in Mark 1:2 is downright foolish!

I know personally of two cases where people tried to imitate Jesus' prolonged fast and the results were disastrous. The first case was a personal friend of mine who lived in Miami. He attempted a forty-day fast. During the third week, he literally went berserk and had to be hospitalized. I'm happy to say that after he was hospitalized, his body and mind began to function properly again, and he's doing fine today. The other case didn't have such a happy ending.

My cousin became a Christian. She was married to an unbeliever. In her eagerness and anxiety over his lost condition, she decided to fast for him until he accepted the Lord. She not only began to fast herself, but she tried to impose fasting upon him. When he came home for dinner, she would put the Bible on his plate and tell him to eat that because that's what he needed. This seems ridiculous, but this is the extreme some of us will go to in trying to save souls instead of trusting God to work in their lives. Well, after a few nights of this, he left her. He wanted to eat and he didn't want any of this nonsense. So he left, and she continued her fast. After so many weeks, she went into a coma and died.

Both of these are true, but tragic, cases of people who tried to imitate what the Lord did. You can't imitate or copy the Lord; you have to be led by Him!

No matter how much I determine I'm going to walk on water

because the Bible says Jesus told Peter to do so, I'm still not going to be able to do it. I can't defy the natural laws of physics with an act of my own will. That's presumption. In fact, the Bible calls it presumptuous sin (Ps. 19:13). Yet, on the other hand, if the Lord bids me to walk on water, and I know beyond a shadow of a doubt down in my spirit (not in my mind) that it's His voice, I believe I could do it. It would be Him leading me, not me trying to copy the acts that He did.

It's the same way with fasting. You can't defy the natural laws of health by an act of your will and win. You won't win. You may do irreparable damage to your body and mind. Jesus said He didn't have a home, "Foxes have holes, and birds of the air have nests; but the Son of man hath not where to lay his head" (Luke 9:58). Does that mean I'm to copy Him in this manner and live on the street or in the forest without having a home? Of course not. Christ is in me. I don't have to copy Him. He's in me, and He's working through me according to the abilities, the talents and the calling He has given to me. I'm the branch and He's the vine. I'm the vessel, and He's the potter. If God wanted us to be Jesus, He would have made us thus, but He made me and He made you and gave us the Spirit of Jesus that He might totally fulfill our destinies according to God's plan. That's the way it is with any aspect of our walk with God, fasting included. He doesn't want carbon copies. He wants individual vessels, each one unique, totally yielded to His purposes in their lives.

Having clarified this, I do not mean to say you're to trust your feelings in the matter of fasting. They can be deceptive. Fasting has to be an act of your will. David said, "I humbled my soul with fasting" (Ps. 69:10 RSV); and Paul said, "I keep under my body, and bring it into subjection" (1 Cor. 9:27). It is very definitely an act of your will and physically and mentally there is a battle to be won. Fasting epitomizes the supremacy of your spirit over your mind and your body, and for this reason there is a tremendous spiritual power released and many other benefits when you fast.

Paul didn't try to copy Jesus and go on a forty-day fast. Yet, it is recorded that he was "in fastings often" (2 Cor. 11:27). This is why I believe that moderate fasting on a somewhat regular basis fulfills the scriptural pattern for our lives today, and complies with the natural laws of good health. By moderate fasting, I mean one to three days. Most fasting recorded in the Scripture was not longer than a day. As I said earlier, I don't believe a person should attempt to fast beyond seven to ten days at any time.

If you have never fasted before, don't attempt to fast for more than one day at a time. After you have conditioned your body to the discipline of fasting, you will be able to fast for longer periods. To attempt a fast beyond one day initially may lead to disappointment and failure because "The spirit indeed is willing, but the flesh is weak" (Matt. 26:41). Be sure to diligently seek the Lord in prayer before attempting any fast beyond three days.

A moderate fast does comply with the natural laws of health for your body in that it allows certain parts of your body to rest, especially the entire digestive system, and it purges your body of impurities, toxic substances, and fat deposits that have built up. Often, when the body is afflicted with a disease such as a fever, our bodies tell us to stop eating so that energy that is usually used on digesting and assimilation of food can be directed to fighting the invading disease. Our appetite often leaves us when sickness is about to strike. Fasting allows our bodies to get rid of the substances that are noᴸ good for us.

As has been stressed throughout this book, when you come off a fast, it's important to comply with sound eating and drinking habits. It's not going to do you much good to purge

140

your body from the effects of wrong eating and then resume eating the same refined carbohydrates and other junk foods. In fact, as the healthful eating and drinking habits you've learned so far become habitual in your life, you'll find it much easier to fast from time to time.

A person who drinks a lot of tea, coffee or chocolate (substances that contain the drug caffeine in them and are definitely not good for you) will often experience headaches on the first day or two of a fast. The same will be true of a person who normally eats a lot of refined sugar products. This happens because your body is experiencing mild withdrawal symptoms from these drugs and unhealthy foods. People who don't use these things in their diets are often not troubled with headaches unless they are having withdrawal from some other food that is equally not good for them. The point is that the more healthful and sound your eating habits, the easier it will be for you to go on a fast and to obtain maximum benefits.

Even with sound eating habits, you must expect your body and mind to be in rebellion at the beginning of a fast. You will experience discomfort. You will experience hunger pangs and thoughts of food, but you can bring those into subjection. Remember a hunger pang only lasts a few minutes and by drinking a glass of water during a hunger pang, you can alleviate it. After two or three days the hunger pang usually subsides. The reason for these discomforts is that your body begins to live on surplus fat, eliminate excess waste, and burn up decaying tissue. You must remember, too, that your body has been conditioned for years to eat so many times a day, all year long, day in and day out. When that conditioned pattern is broken, your body will react. Normally, when you're eating three meals a day, your digestive system converts all carbohydrates, sugars and starches, and a portion of your protein, into glucose—or what is known as blood sugar. This glucose supplies your brain with energy. When you fast, and meals are eliminated, your blood sugar level drops. As a result, you feel uneasy, weaker and sometimes even experience mild nausea. You might also experience depression. You will have bad breath and your tongue will feel coated. The simplest movements of your body may feel like they require a real effort.

These experiences seem to be felt more on the second or third day of a fast as the body is eliminating the stored-up wastes and toxicity that have been in your system for so long. Be sure to rest during these experiences and drink plenty of filtered water which will help flush out many of the impurities. Usually, after the third day or so, you begin to feel renewed strength with only occasional feelings of weakness. Food becomes inconsequential in your thoughts and your body stops craving it. It's at this point, when new strength and vitality come back, that many people make the mistake of deciding to prolong their fasts. This is why I say it is most unwise to continue a fast beyond one week to ten days unless you have direct leading from the Lord. Even if you don't feel like eating, you should begin to at this point, and end your fast.

Some authorities disagree with me on this matter, preferring to let nature take its natural course, but I believe a daily enema is good while fasting. Even though your system is not eliminating the wastes from food, decaying of cells continues to take place and waste material from your entire body is still being funneled into your bowels. I believe it's better to remove these impurities, rather than let them accumulate until after the fast and normal bowel movements begin again with the reentry of food into the system. Don't be alarmed if you don't have a bowel movement after a fast for a day or two. Your entire system has been given a rest and been cleaned out. Give it time to resume its natural order again. It will, and it will then function better than ever.

You may be wondering, with all this physical and emotional discomfort, what are the benefits of fasting? They are many. The primary motives and benefits are spiritual. Prayer and fasting are mighty weapons in our spiritual arsenal. Physically, after the fast is ended, you will feel much better. This way of glorifying God in your body will bring new vigor and health to you. By eliminating the poisons in your system and giving various organs of your body a rest, you will actually begin to feel rejuvenated. Your skin will be clearer. Your eyes will look brighter. You'll feel lighter and have a more buoyant step. And your entire digestive system will feel like new. Some people claim their mental powers improve, and they're able to think more clearly. The benefits of fasting are many and you musι remember too that our heavenly Father has promised to reward us openly when we fast unto him privately. So expect a blessing spiritually and physically, when you fast, because you will always get it.

There's one other benefit of fasting. Each of us has what can be described as a dual nervous system. There is the "sympathetic" nervous system and there is the "parasympathetic" nervous system. These two systems work hand in hand, but often they get out of balance. The sympathetic nervous system is the stimulating part of your nervous system, while the parasympathetic nervous system is the controlling part of your nervous system.

Again, the automobile provides us with a good analogy. Acceleration is like the sympathetic nervous system going into operation. It stimulates the car and makes it go. It motivates and causes action. The brakes and steering mechanism are like the parasympathetic nervous system. They control the thrust that the acceleration provides. Now if your acceleration (your speed and power) is greater than your steering and braking controls, that car will be dangerous to drive. It can get out of control. Conversely, if you've got a braking and steering system designed for a Mack truck and you've got a little Honda engine, that car will be too clumsy to maneuver properly. You must have the right engine balanced with the right braking and steering. The key is balance. Fasting provides a balance between your sympathetic and parasympathetic nervous systems. Your drive and motivation become equally balanced with your controls. This is what helps you to experience a wonderful sense of well-being, a balanced physical and emotional well-being, after a fast.

When you end your fast, you shouldn't eat anything heavy, and guard against overeating. It's very important to slowly reintroduce food into your system after a fast. Your entire digestive system has been resting and been restored. Your stomach has shrunk to about the size of your fist with one hand covering it, so you don't want to gorge it with food. A good way to end your fast is to drink some fruit juice first. Fruit juice is a good source for glucose and will be rapidly assimilated into your system. After that, continue with the order of eating you have learned. (It would be wise to eat acid fruit or cheese for your initial protein instead of meat because they are not as heavy on the stomach.) I would not suggest eating meat for a day or so after a fast of three days. For a fast of a week to ten days refrain from eating meat for at least a couple of days and allow your system to work on lighter foods first. Fasting according to God's natural laws of health is a practical and invigorating method for renewing you—spiritually, emotionally and physically.

In addition to the physical benefits that come to us by fasting there is also a spiritual discipline that results. During His fasting Jesus demonstrated His power over every appetite and desire of mankind. From that time on whenever Satan met Jesus, he knew who had control. His appetite was under control; His desire for possessions was under control; His emotions were under control and not under the dominion of Satan, so that Satan could not tempt Him beyond His power of resistance. Whenever there was a confrontation between them, both always knew who was the master.

You will have trouble rebuking Satan when you do not have every part of your being under control—spirit, soul and body. If you have proven by fasting and disciplining yourself, however, that you are master of your appetites, desires and emotions, you too can cast out devils and you can rebuke and resist Satan when you are tempted. This is the real benefit that comes from fasting. You will know, God will know and Satan will know who is in control of your entire being.

Your body is the temple of the Holy Ghost. God isn't glorified when you are sick, diseased and in a weakened condition through neglect of His natural laws of spiritual, mental and physical health. We're living in a day when there are so many pressures upon God's people, that many Christians give up control of certain areas because they just aren't aware of the provisions the Lord has made for them—through His Word, His divine, natural laws of better health and well-being. God doesn't get any glory when we destroy ourselves emotionally because we're overworking and not spending enough time with our loved ones. He doesn't get any glory when we become sick because we have ignored His natural laws for good physical health. We need to work, but we also need to rest. We need to stop overfeeding ourselves, while at the same time remaining undernourished. Jesus came to give us abundant life (John 10:10), but He won't do for us what we can and must do for ourselves to enter into that abundant living.

As a physician, God has given me the knowledge to help thousands of people to live healthier, happier lives. As a minister of God's Word He has given me a burden for His people that they might experience the abundant living He has blessed me with during my sojourning here on planet earth.

It has not been my intention to place anyone who has read this book under any type of legalistic bondage to a set of rules and regulations, but simply to share the knowledge of my lifelong study of preventive medicine that you might truly become wholly holy.

For free information on how to receive
the international magazine

LOGOS JOURNAL

also Book Catalog

Write: Information - LOGOS JOURNAL CATALOG
Box 191
Plainfield, NJ 07061